Healing Through Exercise

Healing Through Exercise

Scientifically Proven Ways to Prevent and Overcome Illness and Lengthen Your Life

JÖRG BLECH

A MERLOYD LAWRENCE BOOK
LIFELONG BOOKS • DA CAPO PRESS
A Member of the Perseus Books Group

Translation copyright © 2009 by Jörg Blech
Originally published as "Heilen mit Bewegung" by S. Fischer Verlag: Copyright © 2009 by S. Fischer Verlag, Frankfurt am Main. The book was revised and updated for this edition.

Designed by Brent Wilcox
Set in 12 point Minion by the Perseus Books Group

Cataloging-in-Publication data for this book is available from the Library of Congress.

First Da Capo Press edition 2009
ISBN-13: 978-0-7382-1299-9

Published as a Merloyd Lawrence Book by Da Capo Press
A Member of the Perseus Books Group
www.dacapopress.com

Note: The information in this book is true and complete to the best of our knowledge. This book is intended only as an informative guide for those wishing to know more about health issues. In no way is this book intended to replace, countermand, or conflict with the advice given to you by your own physician. The ultimate decision concerning care should be made between you and your doctor. We strongly recommend you follow his or her advice. Information in this book is general and is offered with no guarantees on the part of the authors or Da Capo Press. The authors and publisher disclaim all liability in connection with the use of this book. The names and identifying details of people associated with events described in this book have been changed. Any similarity to actual persons is coincidental.

Da Capo Press books are available at special discounts for bulk purchases in the U.S. by corporations, institutions, and other organizations. For more information, please contact the Special Markets Department at the Perseus Books Group, 2300 Chestnut Street, Suite 200, Philadelphia, PA, 19103, or call (800) 810-4145, ext. 5000, or e-mail special.markets@ perseusbooks.com.

10 9 8 7 6 5 4 3 2 1

To Anke, Hannah, Antonia, and Leo, with love

Our nature consists in motion; complete rest is death
BLAISE PASCAL

CONTENTS

PREFACE

Many diseases can be cured with abstinence and rest, the famous physician Hippocrates decreed more than 2000 years ago. Lately, however, his pronouncement has been called into question. In study after study, physicians now prescribe physical exercise for a whole range of different illnesses— and they see much better results than doctors using conventional medicine.

These results are novel, and exercise hasn't yet been granted the attention it deserves. The marvelous therapeutic effects achieved with exercise are described only in scientific papers scattered throughout the medical literature—and have thus been hidden from many doctors and most laypeople.

This lack of awareness results in poor and often downright bad treatment because patients and physicians alike far too often try to fix medical problems with drugs, high-technology procedures, and simply resting in bed.

This book aims to change that. It's my goal to present the new science of *healing through exercise* for a wide audience. I've researched and written this account in the United States, but have added material from European researchers whenever it was insightful and important.

The new research presented in the following chapters applies to healthy readers as well as to people who have already fallen sick. It turns out that we profit from physical exercise to a much greater degree than doctors have previously believed. In particular, individuals who are middle-aged or elderly are able to stave off illnesses and ailments with dramatic results as soon as they get in motion.

My first research on this subject dates back to the summer of 2005 when I began to work as the science correspondent in the United States for Europe's largest weekly news magazine, *Der Spiegel*. The more I learned about the benefits of exercise, the more I felt the urge to get off my chair, go out—get moving. It became clear to me that it was time to change my life. I started to commute to work using my own muscles. Whether I ride my bicycle or simply walk, I cover eight miles on the local bike path every day. It would be great if the facts and stories I present here moved you in a similar way.

1

The Healing Power of Exercise

At FIRST GLANCE, THE OFFICE OF THE CALIFORNIAN PSYCHIATRIST Wayne Sandler looks just as one might expect: pictures of Sigmund Freud on the wall, tomes on brain anatomy in a glass cabinet, and of course the requisite couch.

But there is one thing that seems rather out of place: two treadmills.

"Patients were always telling me how well they felt when they took proper exercise," says Sandler from his practice on the ninth floor of a building in the affluent Century City district in Los Angeles. But they complained that they never found time or just felt too unwell to practice sports. That's why Wayne Sandler decided to combine his standard therapy sessions with physical exercise.

Around half of Doctor Sandler's depressive or phobic patients bring their sneakers along to appointments. The wiry psychiatrist, who lifts weights or pedals away on a cycling machine every day himself, changes into his black tracksuit. Sandler has set the treadmills up facing each other so that he can look his patients in the eye. All he has to do is switch them on, and the therapy in motion can begin.

Sandler still prescribes medications, such as the fashionable Prozac antidepressant, for some of his patients. But he is convinced that in many cases exercise can deal with chemical imbalances in the brain better than drugs. His clients-cum-jogging partners are very enthusiastic, he reports, and he now prescribes exercise just like a drug: "Movement will be your medicine now—and you need at least 30 minutes of it every day."[1]

Carolyn Kaelin is another believer in the healing power of exercise. A mother of two children, she lives in Boston. In the summer of 2003 she fell ill from breast cancer, at the age of just 42. A course of chemotherapy and five operations including a dual mastectomy couldn't stop Kaelin from going to the gym as often as possible and walking to work every day: "It's the one thing I can do for myself that I know is useful."

Kaelin knows what she's talking about. She is one of America's best-known breast cancer surgeons and runs the Comprehensive Breast Health Center at Brigham and Women's Hospital, part of Harvard Medical School. Seeing her bright smile and sensing her vitality, it's hard to believe the suffering she's been through. But that's what nourishes hope now in the audience of women attending her lectures, with headscarves or a new crop of very short hair.

A growing number of studies, Kaelin tells her fascinated audience, shows that physical exercise can prolong the lives of breast cancer patients and reduce the likelihood of relapses. If diagnosed with breast cancer, the professor recommends women should start a fitness program as soon as possible: "I know it may be the last thing you feel like doing, but I believe it can honestly save your life."[2]

EXERCISE AS MEDICINE

Until now, doctors have usually recommended physical activity and sport as a preventive measure to avoid the outbreak of disease and disorders. But recently, exercise has found its way into the heart of medicine. Psychiatrists and oncologists, orthopedics specialists, dementia researchers, and cardiologists are realizing that physical activity can help people even after they fall ill. In many cases, carefully administered exercise accompanies standard therapies. According to a growing body of evidence, exercise often works better than these therapies. It can make health-promoting cells grow in diseased tissue—and literally turn a disease around.

It is the mind itself, according to the poet Friedrich Schiller, that builds the body. For many years, the medical community thought the opposite was not possible. Neurology textbooks stated that muscle activity could not influence the brain in any way: A mysterious organ, called automatism center, kept the brain's circulation and metabolism at a constant level, the books said, regardless of whether the body was climbing a mountain or dozing in a shady orchard.[3] Compounding this error was the belief that an adult brain could never rejuvenate itself; no new nerve cells were thought to grow after birth. The medical profession held that the brain could only stand still or decline.

Today's brain researchers are correcting that devastating view. The body builds the mind as well as itself. If you exercise your muscles, you practically flood your gray cells with fresh nutrients and growth factors. These make new nerve cells grow. The new cells are easily stimulated and particularly capable of learning. But if we don't make use of them, they die after a few weeks.[4] "Exercise is the strongest known stimulus to grow new nerve cells," says Henriette van Praag, an expert on neurogenesis at the Neuroplasticity and Behavior Unit of the National Institute on Aging in Baltimore.[5] Once nerve cells are produced, mental activity is needed for these newcomers to survive. When used, the neurons are permanently integrated into the brain and able to increase its ability to learn.

That means we can train the brain just like a muscle, at any age. "Fitness training improves neuronal efficiency and performance," says the psychologist Arthur Kramer at the University of Illinois in Urbana-Champaign. "Older brains are a lot more flexible and plastic than we have been led to believe."[6]

No one has to work up much of a sweat to benefit from the healthy effects: People who exert themselves physically for half an hour three times a week, as researchers at Duke University discovered in a comparative study, protect themselves just as effectively against bad moods and attacks of depression as those who take mood enhancers every day.[7] A study led by the University of Melbourne showed that walking for two and a half hours per week improves memory for older people and may stave off dementia.[8]

These encouraging findings are being made because doctors around the world are starting to study and measure the actual effects of physical exercise and evaluate its benefits. Many of these studies show that moderate training can be seen as a form of medicine in its own right, which can be confidently prescribed like a tried and tested drug. Medicine has reached a turning point, say researchers at the University of Copenhagen: The accumulated knowledge on the blessings of exercise "is now so extensive that it has to be implemented."[9]

This paradigm shift to advising activity rather than rest involves the major diseases in particular. Osteoporosis, asthma, osteoarthritis, chronic back pain, and type 2 diabetes, for example, can all be improved and even overcome by exercise. In addition, hyperactive schoolchildren are being prescribed physical activity at playtime instead of pills. Tablets like Viagra can be replaced—by moderate exercise. A long-term study carried out on more than 500 men led researchers to conclude the only behavior that helps impotence patients is regular physical activity.[10]

Exercise also has a therapeutic effect on heart patients. If you raise the number of calories you burn, you reduce the probability of blockages in your coronary arteries. The cardiologist Rainer Hambrecht from the Bremen Heart Centre is studying this phenomenon at the level of single cells. "Patients with stable coronary heart disease," he sums up his findings, "can increase their life expectancy by taking up a sport."

Yet many doctors still recommend rest for various illnesses or even advise patients against any kind of physical activity. Especially for metabolic diseases such as diabetes and osteoarthritis, doing nothing can worsen the patients' quality of life. The more researchers are finding out about these effects, the louder they're calling for a change to the traditional advice for sick people to stay in bed.

"We are getting better, but there is still a long way to go," says Robert Sallis, a family doctor in California and a past president of the American College of Sports Medicine. "Physicians increasingly acknowledge that exercise is good, but I do not think they are trained to think about it as a remedy. They much more quickly pull out their pad and write prescriptions for drugs, and they don't have the training to help their patients to get more active."[11]

Cancer patients in particular are still often advised against physical activity—because doctors believe that that helps them to cope better with the strenuous treatment. But it appears that the opposite is the case.[12] Some physicians are now placing stationary bicycles next to the sickbeds of even seriously ill patients—and they find exercise cheers patients up and gives them back the energy they thought they had lost forever. Physical activity can strengthen the body's own defenses against cancer—and even prolong the life of cancer patients.[13]

Strangely, these exciting findings have hardly made the rounds. The therapeutic value of sport in aftercare for cancer patients appears comparatively unknown and is often rather neglected. Melinda Irwin, a researcher at the Department of Epidemiology and Public Health at Yale School of Medicine in New Haven, says: "The leap has not been made that physicians recommend exercise for cancer patients."[14]

Unfortunately, doctors' advice for patients to rest is often likely to shorten many of the patients' lives. Take heart failure, for example: The physiological processes that cause the problem of weak heart muscles are only made worse if the patient stops taking exercise, on their doctor's advice. Well-informed physicians are now recommending the opposite: According to recent studies, sport can reduce the likelihood of dying from stable chronic heart failure by about 35 percent.[15]

KEEP MOVING TO LIVE LONGER

Researchers have also taken a new look at the effects of inactivity on healthy people. They have shown that office workers who make only minimal use of their muscles put themselves at almost as much risk as smokers. The mortality rate of inactive people is up to one-third higher than that of people who take regular exercise. A 65-year-old who walks less than one mile per day might die seven years earlier than a neighbor of the same age and the same risks otherwise who walks more than two miles per day.[16]

The rule is the same for everyone on the planet: If you engage in regular physical activity and push your muscles, you trigger adaptive processes that have a positive effect on your health. That doesn't just go for sports that revolve around top performance, winning, and losing. It's true for any way we bestir ourselves, including walking and such everyday activities as climbing stairs, cycling, weeding the garden, and cleaning the house. It's this kind of healthy exercise that keeps us young and lengthens our lives, if we keep doing it in later life. The reward for burning an extra 500 to 2000 kilocalories a week is living longer; the mortality risk is 28 percent lower for 60- to 69-year-olds, and 37 percent for 70- to 84-year-olds.[17]

Evolutionary physiologists like Frank Booth from the University of Missouri in Columbia say it's a fallacy to believe that physical inactivity does no further harm, as long as you keep a steady weight and eat sensibly. Modern human beings are still genetically programmed for life as hunters and gatherers because our genetic composition has hardly changed in the

10,000 years since the Stone Age. Back then, our ancestors were in top athletic form every day, looking for food, hunting wild animals, and building shelters. Those who weren't able to keep up simply died out. Those who survived passed down the biological equipment needed under these conditions over the millennia. That means we all have perfectly functioning bodies—but only as long as we take exercise on a daily basis.

Presently, however, a large part of the world's population makes a living in ways for which their genetic inheritance was never designed: Billions of people spend most of their lives sitting, at work and after.

We do of course live much longer lives than the cavemen, thanks to improved hygiene, obstetrics, and antibiotics. But "the average office worker would be much more healthy," according to the American evolutionary biologists Randolph Nesse and George Williams, "if he or she spent the day digging clams or harvesting fruit in scattered tall trees."[18]

Because the biochemical cycles get sluggish in inactive bodies, fats in the blood tend to form gallstones more often, for example. People who don't take exercise have their gall bladders removed more often than the rest of the population. And because digestion slows down in bodies that don't move much, the period of contact with carcinogenic substances in our food is lengthened; inactive people have a 50 percent higher risk of contracting bowel cancer. Even the genes became affected because being lazy appears to make us genetically old before our time. Researchers in Newark, New Jersey, and London found that pieces of DNA called telomeres shorten faster in physically inactive people, making them prone to quicker cellular aging.[19]

Frank Booth puts most diseases of modern life down to the fact that our metabolisms are going off course because of chronic lack of activity. He and other scientists recommend a minimum of 30 minutes of moderate exercise a day—walking or swimming, for example. Everything below that is defined as inactive. "Without that threshold of physical activity expected by our genomes," says Booth, "physiological dysfunction is likely to occur from pathological gene expression, eventually leading to chronic health conditions."[20]

If this sounds gradual, and not that threatening, put it this way: The body of anyone who doesn't take at least half an hour of exercise every day is in a state of emergency. Pathological processes are constantly taking place in the cells and tissues, and it's only a matter of time until irritations and complaints break out.

According to the evolutionary biologists, we have to rethink the old view of exercise: movement is by no means just a useful added way to improve our health. In fact, it is absolutely necessary for the human body to work normally. That goes for all ages: Children can develop their mental abilities properly only if they do enough running, jumping, and physical playing as well. Motor and cognitive skills develop in unison and stimulate each other within the brain. Researchers in the field of neuroanatomy at the University of Bielefeld sum up what that means for parents, children, and teachers: "Learning needs movement."

The new findings suddenly put what we think of the aging process in a different light: many of the changes are to a great extent the result of inactivity.[21] We spend vast amounts of money on the products of the antiaging industry, but so far all the pills, hormones, live cell injections, vitamin cures, and orthomolecular procedures have been an abject failure. But don't despair: A fountain of youth is at hand—but it just takes a little effort. Only regular physical activity can slow up the biological aging process. In other words, being active is the only way not to look old.

We don't age chronologically but biologically. If we keep our bodily functions vital, we can slow down or stop the biological aging process—over decades. That's practically a law of nature, and you and I can make it work for us.

Of course, physical exercise can never guarantee that an individual won't get sick. The author James Fixx remodeled long-distance running as "jogging" and popularized it around the world—only to collapse and die at the age of 52 while out on a jog on a lonely country road. However, atherosclerosis was running in his family, and he might have died earlier without picking up the habit of exercising.

No one is claiming we can literally run away from sickness. The Norwegian Grete Waitz won the New York City Marathon nine times and has recently been battling cancer. The cyclist Lance Armstrong contracted testicular cancer after becoming the world road race champion. These stories illustrate that fate and bad luck also play a role in disease, especially tumors.

We all know the feeling: whenever we come down with an illness, we always look for explanations, for reasons why it got so far. But doctors have long since found evidence that the course of health disorders is influenced by not only genetic and environmental factors, but also by pure coincidence.[22] By the time Lance Armstrong was diagnosed with cancer, he had metastases in the whole of his body and brain. The doctors estimated his chance of survival at below 50 percent. Armstrong himself puts the fact that he was still healed and made a spectacular recovery down to "a lucky coincidence."

But at the same time, the likelihood of many healthy decades of life can be improved by living an active lifestyle. Epidemiological studies indicate one factor again and again: Daily physical activity is linked with a lower risk of cardiovascular diseases, strokes, loss of memory, depression, type 2 diabetes, obesity—and with a longer life. It also reduces the risk of breast and bowel cancer. There is no doubt: If we could put the positive effects of moderate exercise in a bottle, we'd all take a good swig from it every morning. Canadian doctors reported that the elixir is even stronger and more effective than previously assumed. "Recent investigations have revealed even greater reductions in the risk of death from any cause and from cardiovascular disease. For example, being fit or active was associated with a greater than 50 percent reduction in risk."[23]

Ninety percent of over-50s would benefit from regular training—and the good news is, it works just as well if we take it slowly. It doesn't always have to be jogging—even brisk walking has proven effective.

OUTDATED ADVICE

While part of the medical community is now hailing a new era of "active medicine," many doctors remain skeptical about exercise, as physician Annette Becker from the University of Marburg remarks with astonishment. There is now "highest evidence for the effectiveness of exercise in the prevention and treatment of chronic diseases, and for the ineffectiveness or even detrimental effects of bed-rest," she comments. "But many doctors still often advise their patients to stay in bed for long periods, which can—as in the treatment of chronic pain—worsen the patients' prognosis."[24]

Experts at the University of Hamburg also find it "amazing how little many doctors know about these things."[25] Because of this ignorance, patients—possibly in the thousands at any given time—are simply being wrongly treated. Let's look at patients with back pain. Physicians are all too keen to carry out expensive diagnosis procedures such as computer tomography and MRI scans. These rarely produce pathological findings but do mean high income for the doctors. The patients are sent away with prescription drugs—and often do not receive the physiotherapy they actually need or, more important, any help for changing their lifestyles in the long term. Patients diagnosed with mild high blood pressure are usually prescribed expensive medication; "Doctors seldom think of prescribing a program of moderate stamina training."[26]

In defense of the physicians, all this is the exact opposite of what must have been learned at medical school. What we now know is wrong was considered right back when current doctors were students. Sending sick people to bed made everyone happy. The whole way of thinking, the medical practice of the time, was founded on the basic conviction that patients would find salvation in physical rest.

Many of the experienced doctors who now run large practices or hospital departments went to medical school at a time when heart attack patients were still ordered to spend four to six weeks in bed. Some older doctors may remember a time when patients were even strapped down to keep them still. Not that long ago they were of the opinion that our hearts only had a limited number of beats, according to the motto: "Use up those beats by racing your heart with exercise, and you shorten your life span."[27]

In his classic book *The Structure of Scientific Revolutions,* the American historian Thomas Kuhn describes why it's always so hard for new findings to take the place of old ideas in science.[28] Fundamental new ideas are initially disdained because they undermine scientists' previous work and reveal that this work is wrong or even foolish. Eventually some scholars adopt the new theory, whereas others stubbornly refuse to alter their positions. The latter gradually die out until their views are entirely forgotten.

When it comes to exercise as medicine, we have not yet reached that turning point: "The paradigm shift is in flux, but has not yet been realized in this short period of time."[29] There are signs that it might take a while yet until the breakthrough. Even now, medical training barely addresses the links between regular activity, fitness, and disease.

But it's not just the medical profession that hasn't caught on to the healing power of exercise. We laypersons have also failed to recognize its benefits. When our grandparents were growing up, most people in industrial societies never reached old age, worn out by dangerous physical labor on the factory floor or relentless household labor. Their grandchildren now live in what we could call sitting societies. We are the first generation to face the opposite challenge: We may grow old before our time and die young if we don't get enough exercise.

2

The Dangers of Going to Bed

A MEDICAL TREATMENT OFTEN BEGINS BY PUTTING A PATIENT TO bed. Many of us have already had this experience: having barely arrived at a hospital, we are asked to remove our street clothes, put on a skimpy gown or pair of pajamas, and go to bed. The size of a hospital is measured by the number of beds it has, and the severity of an illness is determined by the number of days a patient stays in bed. And whether or not we like a physician depends on that doctor's "bedside manners." A good doctor sits down by the patient's bed and listens.

An example of such medical tact is depicted in Pablo Picasso's painting *Science and Charity* from 1897. A bearded doctor is taking the pulse of an exhausted patient; he represents science. On the other side of the bed, a nun faces the patient; she represents charity. Picasso's creation shows a vision of how bed rest should be, says the general practitioner Annette Becker, of the University Hospital in Marburg, Germany. She believes that rest means "not only immobilization but also care, gentleness and protection for an individual who is burdened by disease."[1]

A DANGEROUS PRESCRIPTION

Over the years, bed rest has been prescribed in far more coercive ways. The American neurologist Silas Weir Mitchell (1829–1914) introduced something he called the "rest cure." For Mitchell, the best treatment for individuals suffering from neurasthenia as well as hysteria was to confine them to bed for six to eight weeks. During this agonizing period, some patients were not even allowed to turn their bodies without support. This type of immobilization soon was taken up by virtually the entire medical world, especially for individuals said to be hysterical. During their detainment, these poor souls were not allowed to receive visitors and, in order to avoid any distress, they were always cared for by the same nurse. The patients were forbidden to use their own hands for washing, and their nurses fed them a diet consisting of especially fatty dairy products. Mitchell actually reported many recoveries: as soon as he allowed his patients to go back into everyday life, they were usually more than willing to flee this sickbed.

The perils of bed rest, however, have been known to more enlightened physicians. Richard Asher (1912–1969), who worked at the Central Middlesex Hospital in England, was making his rounds one day when he came across a remarkable case of bed rest. "In a chronic ward of which I once had charge I found a lady who had been in bed for 17 years with a diagnosis of nervous debility and whitlow," Asher reported in the *British Medical Journal*. "She had survived this remarkable hibernation with little damage, and though she was very upset when I ordered her up she became a different person when she was fully ambulant."[2]

There is a long tradition of doctors exercising power over individuals by confining them to bed. In the novel *The Magic Mountain*, soon after the young Hans Castorp arrives at the International Sanatorium Berghof, where he wanted to visit his cousin, he is ordered to bed. "Now, Castorp, we'll stick you into bed and see if a couple of weeks' rest will sober you up," the physician Herr Hofrat Behrens tells him. "As if 'lie down' isn't just as good a word of command as 'stand up'!"[3]

The French writer Jules Romains recounts in his satire on medical quackery, *Knock*, the story of a country doctor named Knock who, by inventing outlandish diseases, turns a whole mountain village into a hospital. This disease-monger tells his first patient, a lady in black, "Go to bed when you get home. In a room where you can be alone as much as possible. Close the shutters and draw the curtains so the light won't bother you. Don't let anyone talk to you." The doctor orders a full week of this isolation, after which he will reconsider the case. Knock says: "If you are strong and full of life it will mean that things aren't as bad as they seem. If, on the other hand, you're weak and drowsy, have a hard time getting up, then there's no doubt about it and we'll have to start the treatment."[4]

Over the course of the story, the woman falls sick and confirms Dr. Knock's case for treatment. Findings from real-life research explain why this outcome is likely. After spending just a few days in bed, our muscles start to waste away and a whole range of undermining effects sets in. Being immobilized can bring more harm to our health than the ailments, which sent us to bed in the first place.

"Bed Rest: A Potentially Harmful Treatment Needing More Careful Evaluation": this is the title Australian doctors chose for a paper they published in the medical journal *The Lancet*.[5] They had carried out a review of the scientific literature on the use of bed rest in treating various illnesses. In 24 trials that looked into bed rest following a medical procedure, the review revealed that none of the outcomes improved significantly. In eight of these trials, bed rest actually worsened the outcome—for example following lumbar puncture, cardiac catherization, and spinal anesthesia.

Fifteen of these trials examined bed rest as a primary remedy, and in these studies the results were even more sobering. While not a single group of patients got better, in nine diagnostic groups the health of the involved patients on average actually got *worse*. This was the case after acute low back pain, childbirth, high blood pressure during pregnancy, heart attack, and acute infectious hepatitis.

The authors of the review article were amazed that so many members of the medical profession were clinging to the ritual of putting patients to bed, even though the bed-rest trials they reviewed had been published for quite some time. "Ideas about bed rest seem so entrenched that medical practice has been slow to change—even when faced with evidence of ineffectiveness."[6]

Researchers at the Yale School of Medicine have come to the conclusion that the effect of bed rest is especially detrimental to people age 70 or older. According to their study in the *Journal of the American Medical Association*, the risk of developing a disability within a month of hospitalization was elevated more than 60-fold.[7] In many cases, the physical condition of older people staying in a hospital deteriorates so dramatically that they never return home and instead must be transferred directly to a managed-care facility.

There are only a few researchers studying the phenomenon of being bedridden. The nursing scientist Angelika Zegelin at the University Witten/Herdecke in Germany is one of them. In an unusual study, Zegelin went into an elderly care home and conducted interviews with 12 men and 20 women who dwelled there. These residents were of sound mind but had been bedridden for up to four years. Zegelin wanted to find out: Why did they end up in such a sad situation?

According to her findings, the disastrous scenario leading to the state of being bedridden unfolds in five distinct steps.[8] It often begins when a person develops what Zegelin calls a "physical instability." The individual is actually healthy, but at one point in the life refrains, for whatever reason, from physical activity. This voluntary inactivity may not appear harmful but can have such a deep effect that some people will eventually end up in a nursing home. A survey among 50 residents in one such residential home revealed that 75 percent of its occupants never played sports in their adult lives.[9]

The conversion from being sedentary to being totally immobile, the second stage, is then usually triggered by an accident or a similar event. This incident can be a fall—but it may result solely from the *fear* of falling. In many instances, a stay in a hospital became the starting point for further physical decline. At least, this is what Zegelin heard time and again during her survey interviews. Many of her subjects stated they "just stayed in bed during their hospital stay, and after one week they were already unable to get up."[10]

This triggers the third phase, which is the one of continuous immobility. The individual in question walks only a few steps and for most of the day is simply lying in bed or sitting in an armchair. If he or she still lives at home, then he or she is looked after by a nursing service.

At this stage, some exercise would still be very helpful—but typically no one is around to help mobilize the ill person. According to a survey among 70 residents in one nursing home, 66 percent of them had fewer than two hours of physical motion per week, and a third of the residents did not move at all. The situation was partly worsened by an unfortunate misunderstanding. Some of the older persons refrained from leaving their beds because they did not want to cause more work for the nurses who appeared to be overburdened, especially on the weekends. Conversely, many nurses assumed they were being kind to the frail residents by not disturbing their rest. Thus, unsurprisingly, the survey concludes that there is "widespread physical inactivity in nursery homes."[11]

Many older people and invalids who are looked after in their own homes are also hardly able to leave their beds. A caregiver from a nursing service might show up two or three times per day, but they usually are in a hurry and leave again after only 20 to 30 minutes. The ailing individuals may ask to be guided to a chair, but once the nurses are gone, they must sit there for hours, until the next nursing shift arrives, at which point a caregiver can help them back to bed. Thus, most people interviewed by Zegelin vowed not to leave their beds in the first place.

By now, the fourth stage of the decline is reached: confinement to only one spot. Patients resign themselves to the dim prospect of spending every minute in the same spot, with the exception of using the bathroom, for which they need assistance.

This physical decline is usually associated with a cognitive one. At the beginning of their immobile existences, these ailing individuals tend to watch television, but that becomes too boring after a while. Reading often becomes impossible because they lack the muscle strength to hold books. Visitors are rare, creating a condition of mental vacuity. "The immobile patients are caught in an eventless world and subsequently they lose their sense for time. Months and years dwindled, being fixed to one place all the time made the concept of time meaningless," observes Zegelin.

Eventually, the patients slide into the fifth and last phase: they are permanently bedridden. They depend on diapers, and they will never again use their legs.

One would like to believe that physicians take measures to avoid such dramatic declines. However, according to Zegelin's survey, it was both well-intentioned advice, as well as medically motivated arrangements, that contributed to these unfortunate circumstances. In the interviews, many of the residents reported being admonished by doctors and nurses to take it easy and to rest their bodies: "If you have another fall, it's all over for you!"

Furthermore, the transfer into a special nursing bed added to the patients' physical immobilization. These beds are often fenced with bars and, because of very thick mattresses, are grotesquely high. When Zegelin asked the residents of the retirement home, "Since when were you actually confined to bed?" too often she heard a revealing answer: "Since they put me in this special bed."

WASTING AWAY IN OUTER SPACE

Scientists first became aware of the importance for patients to keep moving due to an accidental finding from the Second World War, when beds in sick bays and nurses were scarce. Acting from necessity, doctors released the injured and the sick earlier than usual—often resulting in better healing successes and fewer complications. After the war, this approach lived on in U.S. military hospitals, and medical personnel were taught that the consequences of bed rest are often worse than the original injury.[12]

The next hint came from space research. When the United States decided to send astronauts to the moon, it became crucial to understand how zero-gravity conditions would affect a human body confined for many days to a tiny space capsule. Thus, in 1966, the National Aeronautics and Space Administration (NASA) initiated a remarkable endeavor that became known as the Dallas Bed Rest and Training Study.[13] In a Dallas hospital, five young and healthy men were ordered to stay in bed for three weeks. Like the unfortunate patients in Dr. Silas Weir Mitchell's ward, these human guinea pigs were not allowed to move their bodies at all. To avoid weight gain, they were kept on a low-calorie diet. They were allowed to take one shower the whole time and were pushed to the bathroom in a wheelchair. After 21 days, the five men were examined—and it turned out they were physical wrecks. Their ability to consume oxygen was reduced by 28 percent, and when two of the subjects were asked to run on a treadmill, they fainted.

WHILE THE BODY RESTS

We don't fully understand the effects of immobilization on the body, but the findings doctors have gathered in the past 50 years show a broad physical decline. As soon as we spend too much time under the covers, almost every part of the body starts to waste away.

Connective Tissue and Joints

The flexible parts of the body—like joints, tendons, ligaments, muscles, and skin—ordinarily move often, allowing them to function properly. When the freedom of these movements is constrained, these parts shrink. This reaction, known as contracture, can be seen within eight hours of rest: After a night of sleep, some joints and muscles are stiff. While stretching intuitively in the morning, we reverse this early symptom of rest.

Bones

Our bones might appear stable, solid, and hard, but bone tissue is a dynamic structure constantly changing itself. After each stimulus from outside—if we carry a weight or perform push-ups—bone tissue is added, reorganized, or broken down. But as soon as a person takes to bed, bones start to lose calcium, which shows up through increased levels of calcium in the urine after only a few days of bed rest. Scientists have measured this loss and found that 1.54 grams of calcium are excreted per week. This flushing, in turn, increases the risk of kidney stones and of calcification in tissues. This loss of calcium affects the stability of bones. An underused skeleton can soon become crumbly and fragile. People confined to bed for three weeks double their risk of breaking a hip.[14]

Skin

Resting in bed curtails blood flow in the skin tissues. In those areas where the skin does not cover soft tissue but spans directly across a bone, it gets highly compressed. This compression restricts the blood flow in the skin tissue, which is incrementally dissolved, dies off, and turns into a festering sore prone to inflammation.

Muscle

A given muscle is only as strong as it needs to be and is highly adapted to its usual tasks. Thus, given nothing to do, a muscle will start wasting away, losing roughly one-eighth of its strength during one week of physical inactivity. Such atrophy also occurs when we have to carry an arm or leg in a cast; after the plaster is removed, it is amazing to see how stiff and short the unused muscles have become. The voluntary disuse of our body has a similar effect. When a muscle exerts less than 20 percent of its maximum strength, it starts to shrink. In the case of absolute bed rest, the body loses eight grams of protein every day. The back pain that often appears after a few days of bed rest is actually triggered by the fact that stomach muscles, as well as the muscles lining the backbone, are wasting away. Thus the medical tradition of prescribing bed rest to heal back pain seems downright absurd.

Urinary Passages

The renal pelvis drains because of gravity. If a person is lying in a horizontal position all the time, the accumulating urine cannot properly run off, and the fluid is retained in parts of the kidney, in the calyxes. This in turn poses a risk of developing kidney stones and infections.

Lungs

Another problem for people who remain immobile for long periods is that mucus starts to accumulate in certain areas of the lungs, leading to a condition called local atelectasis. As a result, air cannot move properly through the affected areas and, subsequently, the number of deep breaths a person can take decreases. Even people initially in good health before becoming bedridden risk developing atelectasis and lung infections.

Cardiovascular System

Like every other muscle in the body, the heart shrinks as soon as it lacks sufficient work. The Dallas Bed Rest and Training

Study[15] revealed that after three weeks of rest, the heart's stroke volume decreases by 25 percent, and the size of the heart shrinks by 11 percent. In addition, the risk of suffering an embolism rises, as the blood cannot circulate as usual. A thrombus can emerge and can cause a sudden death by blocking a vessel.

Sex and Reproduction

Physical inactivity decreases the production of the male hormone testosterone and dampens the libido. Also, fewer sperm are produced in the testes.

Digestion

When a person lacks movement, the peristalsis usually needed to move the food through the guts slows down. This can lead to digestive problems and constipation.

Psychological Effects of Immobility

At one point, NASA also kept young male test subjects in bed for as much as five weeks, which caused a whole range of mental and sensory problems. These brave men developed sleeping disorders, anxiety, and hostility to the people around them. In addition, there were hints that the physical passivity impaired their senses. Their capability to hear, see, and taste diminished.[16]

Another long-term psychological effect is commonplace in hospitals. As soon as people are admitted, many of them abandon their autonomy and slip into the role of the passive patient. Whenever a doctor or nurse appears, patients act in a servile way and readily abide to every procedure. Other people now control many aspects of their life: what they eat, when they sleep, and when visitors are allowed. The lack of intellectual stimulation leads to a dull state of mind. A stay in a clinic can thus mark a sharp decline in cognitive abilities. Nursing scientists aptly call it "the downswing of the IQ in the hospital."[17] Consequently, after being released from a hospital, a surprisingly high number of people must struggle to go back to their normal lives. As the American physician Paul Corcoran concluded: "Small wonder that many patients have trouble resuming independent management and decision making after prolonged bed rest."[18]

Pain and Rest: A Vicious Circle

Patients being treated because of neurological injuries suffer more often from chronic pain when they—or their affected body part—are immobilized following the treatment. Less well-understood disorders like fibromyalgia and fibrositis also appear connected with the level of physical activity a person maintains. Attacks of pain tend to start during periods without exercise, when the body is in a depleting mode called "deconditioning."

Often a person experiencing pain gets caught in a vicious cycle, cautions Annette Becker: "As soon as the patients feel the pain they start to take it easy. In the beginning, the rest admittedly leads on to some pain relief, but in the long run it gives rise to deconditioning—which, in turn, makes the pain worse. This increase of pain adds to the urge to take it easy. Eventually, the rest becomes the reason for being sick and the sickness becomes the reason for the rest—the pain is likely to become chronic."[19]

PREMATURE AGING

The decline a person suffers in the course of a bed rest of several weeks is, in effect, occurring right now in wide sections of the larger population, albeit distributed across many years in the lives of people. In middle age, around their 40th birthday, many people adopt a passive and sedentary way of life. They never walk their children to school and always use a car for simple errands. The more they sit, the faster their bodily composition changes. While muscles shrink, fat cells get bigger.

In 1988, the physician Irwin Rosenberg of Tufts University in Boston came up with a name for an eerie phenomenon: "sarcopenia" (from the Greek words *sarx*, meaning "flesh," and *penia*, or "deficiency"). People suffering from sarcopenia usually walk extremely slowly and have a reduced bone density. They have a weak grip, are prone to falls, and are often unable to control urination and defecation. Their condition is, in a word, tragic. As Rosenberg states: "The more [the potential sarcopenia victims] sit around, fail to exert themselves, and are waited upon by others, the greater the amount of their body's muscle mass that is replaced by fat. This insidious weakening of body structure and gradual loss of functional capacity then becomes a good excuse for continuing the pattern of immobility."[20] But those affected may think it perfectly normal that they hardly have any physical strength. This, they may declare, is nothing but a natural symptom of old age.

This attitude could not be more dangerous. Such a decline of fitness and bodily control is caused by the fact that muscles haven't been used properly in years. Gradually, the physiological changes mimic the rapid degeneration caused by complete bed rest. In both instances the body's ability to process oxygen, its aerobic capacity, dwindles. While the stroke capacity of the heart decreases, blood pressure increases. The concentration of red blood cells decreases, but that of cholesterol increases. The ability of blood to coagulate, thus healing wounds, is hampered. Sarcopenia and complete bed rest shape the body and the metabolism in strikingly similar ways: The proportion of fat grows at the cost of the muscular system. Calcium is flushed away, and the outer substance of the bones thins. The capability to utilize blood sugar is impaired, and the average body temperature drops. The level of male sex hormones drops, the production of sperm slows down, and the libido—the desire to have sex—is also impaired.

With both long-term physical inactivity and short-term bed rest, fewer neurotransmitters like dopamine and serotonin are active in the brain. The sense of hearing fades, as well as the ability to sleep. The sense of taste is slowly desensitized. Memory becomes worse.

For most people, all these changes arrive over the course of years. For the most part, however, this decline is not caused by the phenomenon of aging but simply by the permanent disuse of the body in the course of those years.

Every sedentary person can demonstrate that this is true because these multiple symptoms of degradation and decomposition will be reversed as soon as a person gets in motion again. That is the good news of this sobering chapter: Even degenerating cells, organs, and tissues can recover. If they are stimulated to move, they will renew themselves, and will do so at every age of a person's life.

3

Unemployed Bodies, New Diseases

IN 1961, PHYSICIANS HANS KRAUS AT NEW YORK UNIVERSITY AND Wilhelm Raab at the University of Vermont College of Medicine wrote of an alarming trend:[1]

> We as physicians, have come to accept as normal what even a century ago might well have been looked upon as below normal, abnormal, or even sick. We blandly accept the fact that men and women in their late thirties cannot run, that they are overweight, that they might have to "watch their hearts," that they need diets, and that they have an assortment of minor or major orthopedic aches and pains. . . .
>
> On the other hand, we consider as supernormal or as freakishly exceptional people whose physical activities approximate those of past generations of less mechanized countries. We consider the low pulse rate of an athlete as something unusual. . . . We are surprised at the relatively low muscular tension, the spontaneous weight control, the better muscle strength and flexibility, the greater breathing capacity and the high fatigue level of the well-trained, not over-trained, athlete, and we settle back comfortably to our daily

sedentary routines after having declared such people un-usual, as indeed they are.[1]

Kraus and Raab described an emerging ailment produced by lack of exercise—the hypokinetic disease—at the same time such revealing terms as "disuse atrophy" and "untrained heart" entered medical dictionaries. Doctors initiated studies asking whether there might be a correlation between physical inactivity and the rate of heart disease. Their conclusions: people with physically demanding jobs were three to four times *less* likely to die from a heart attack. Forty years ago, this outcome caused a sensation: "It is not labor that damages the coronary arteries and the heart—but the lack of labor."[2]

Lack of exercise was found to upset crucial bodily functions and to turn "sleep disorders and impairments of digestion into the most frequent ailments of our time," said Harald Mellerowicz, a sports physician in Berlin. In a blend of cynicism and wrath, he cautioned: "The muscles of the torso are no longer able to give it natural support. Weak and bad postures, degenerations of the spine and of the ribcage develop, with impact on the bloodstream and the respiratory system. This bad posture is not only unattractive but also triggers a whole chain of additional impairments affecting development, health and performance."[3]

STUCK IN OUR CHAIRS

These harsh words, published in 1967, had little effect. No generation has ever moved as little as today's inhabitants of the United States and other Western nations. Experts at the World Health Organization have classified 60 percent of the world's population as sedentary; 41 percent do not even have two hours of moderate exercise per week; 17 percent are completely inactive. It is estimated that 2 million people die from illnesses caused by lack of exercise, among them cardiovascular disease, breast cancer, and type 2 diabetes. In the United States, treatment for sedentary citizens costs 75 billion dollars every year.[4]

However, most people do not consciously decide to be lazy. In general terms, they are yielding to the manifold temptations of the modern world. Though we do not act to avoid them, the hazards are well known. In the 1950s, television sets conquered American households, and gasoline was so cheap then that families, instead of walking, took to road trips on the weekends. Today, there is less need for physical exercise at work, at home, or during recreation, to the point where, as William Haskell at the Stanford University School of Medicine puts it, we can speak of its "non-existence in industrialized and urbanized societies."[5] Haskell himself is deeply worried.

In the United States, children grow up in a world that leaves no time and no room for physical activities. For most of the baby boomers, it was common either to walk or to ride a bicycle to school. In these days, kids are moved around in minivans, and teachers have a hard time advocating walking days. Once in school, students will rarely be challenged physically because many school systems struggle to finance a physical education program worthy of the name. At recess, video games and other gadgets have taken the role balls and skipping ropes used to occupy. The idle members of generation XXL spend their youths indoors, and they would rather travel online than by foot. Granted that some ten-year-olds design impressive Web pages, but many have difficulties climbing, jumping, or pitching a ball. According to Nielsen Media Research data, the average child or adolescent watches an average of nearly three hours of television per day. This figure does not include time spent watching videotapes or playing video games; one 1999 study actually found that children spend an average of six hours and 32 minutes per day with various media combined.[6] No wonder there is literally no time left for playing outdoors.

The abandonment of exercise is a global trend affecting not only kids growing up in American suburbia but also youngsters living in walkable areas of Europe. Wilhelm Niebling has a doctor's office in the idyllic Black Forest. As he puts it: "Many children in our town are not able to balance backwards."

We hardly realize the subtle ways in which digital technologies reduce the amount of exercise we get at work. To start with, often workers no longer have a real need to leave their houses in the first place. Thanks to cell phones, Internet access, faxes, and e-mail, more people can work from their home. And even if an employee finds her way to the office, there she need not leave her cubicle. She can communicate by phone and e-mail with every colleague. Writing, copying, and sending a document can be done without leaving her chair. The automatic redial function on phones reduces even the amount of energy needed to hit the numbers. Over the course of days or weeks, these effects seem to be negligible for our well-being.

In the course of months and years, these small effects make a big difference. To illustrate this point, William Haskell offers the example of an initially slim white-collar worker weighing 60 to 70 kilograms (130 to 150 pounds).[7] Imagine, says Haskell, that the worker had the following choices: He could print all his documents; pick them up at the printer; and personally bring them, like an office boy, to the relevant colleagues. In this case he would rise from his chair once per hour and walk slowly for two minutes. Alternatively, he could send all his documents by e-mail, and he would thus sit all the time. In the latter case, the energy consumption would be decreased by an amount equaling 500 grams of fat per year. That is to say sending e-mails gives rise to an insidious obesity—after ten years the worker will be five kilograms fatter. If the same man walks one kilometer every morning, he may make up for this. However, if he keeps his food intake, but stops his morning strolls, he will gain two kilograms within one year.[8]

OFF THE CHARTS

Not only do people get bigger in wealthy countries like the United States, Kuwait, or Australia, but the wealthy classes in poorer states like Thailand do as well. By now, there are more overweight people living on this planet than there are individuals who have a weight once thought to be normal. However, there is no clear boundary defining the line at which excess weight should be considered a pathology. The Body Mass Index as used in most official guidelines serves only as an approximate guide.[9] If a person arrives at a number between 25 and 30, he or she is overweight, according to the World Health Organization. If the BMI is 30 or higher, the person is obese.

Even though experts disagree whether or not these definitions are too strict, there is no doubt that humans are getting bigger. In 1970, male Americans were on average 8.7 kilograms heavier than men of the same age and height who were examined in 1863. The British army increasingly has had problems finding slim recruits. Earlier this decade, only one-third of 16-year-olds met their requirements, whereas two-thirds were too heavy. In 2006, the army relaxed the rule. Since then, men with a BMI of up to 32 may be recruited; the old cutoff was a BMI of 28.

Our modern habits produce human bodies that were unknown in the Stone Age. In a special clinic for obese adolescents in 2000, I met a boy named Paul. During the first 15 years of his life he put on an average of 820 grams every month. When I interviewed him, he stood five feet and ten inches high and weighed 347.5 pounds—more than half of his body consisted of fat.[10] In the natural world a physiology like this is rare, apart from humans. In summer, the bar-tailed godwit gorges on clams in the estuaries of the Alaskan coast, until fat makes up 55 percent of its body weight. Then, however, the brave bird sets forth on a journey that will take it across the Pacific Ocean to New Zealand. Its fat serves as a fuel tank on an exciting journey that lasts four or five days.[11]

Humans with such enormous padding, by contrast, develop debilitating symptoms and can even become unable to move without assistance. Paul, the student, was suffering from ailments for which he should have been too young. The boy, at age 15, had a fatty liver, and his blood pressure was so high that he was frequently bleeding from his nose. In his body the level of uric acid molecules was dramatically elevated—a sure harbinger of gout. Fat masses constricted Paul's neck so that he couldn't breathe properly while asleep, and his nighttime respiration occasionally went into hiatus. Meanwhile Paul's feet were under immense pressure so that he was walking like a duck on his flatfeet. His shoes were two sizes bigger than they would have been at a normal weight.

In the United States, there is no shortage of freakish stories about people grown so big they can't move. Now in Europe similar tales are making the rounds. In the city of Hamburg, firefighters had to respond to a call from a woman in diabetic shock. She weighed 250 kilograms and wouldn't fit through her door. The firefighters lifted her with a crane from her balcony on the fourth floor. In the city of Düsseldorf authorities have purchased special ambulance cars for such heavy cases: They have heavy duty stretchers and hydraulic ramps.

In American amusement parks, such as Sea World in San Diego, it has become part of the daily routine for some visitors to be too big and heavy to walk through the park. They leave their cars at the spots reserved for disabled persons close to the entrance. Having covered the short distance from their car to the ticket booth, they sit down on electric scooters that take them around. The Israeli company Afikim Electric Mobilizers is one of the suppliers in this market. Originally, its model was designed to carry two or three elderly people with mobility problems. Due to heavy demand from overweight Americans, however, the company has supersized the scooter by upgrading the motor and replacing a two-person bench with a single bucket seat. It can now carry a driver weighing up to 500 pounds.[12]

Airlines, on the other hand, consume more jet fuel due to the increased weight of their customers, and they even must deal with passengers who need two seats but just want to pay for one. On a flight from England to California a young woman suffered from internal bleeding because an obese passenger next to her squeezed her. It wasn't until the victim threatened to sue the airline that she received a compensation of 13,000 British pounds.

Many scientists trace the global spreading of obesity to overeating. However, in the United States the average intake of calories remained roughly the same between 1909 and 1970, and even appears to have slightly shrunk since then. Nonetheless, U.S. citizens have put on a lot of weight because they burn fewer calories through physical exercise.[13]

Nobody knows exactly how the human energy balance looked a few centuries ago. It is estimated that hunter-gatherers burned an average of 1000 kilocalories per day to move their bodies. At the same time, they ate food containing 3000 kilocalories—this is a ratio of 3 to 1. In our time, a sedentary American actually eats less food; his intake amounts to 2400 kilocalories. But he burns only 300 kilocalories per day—this is a ratio of 8 to 1. This mismatch leads to an excess of 100 kilocalories per day—a principal reason for the obesity seen in today's societies.

4

Walking Off Diabetes

In 2006, A GROUP OF RESEARCHERS GATHERED IN MELBOURNE, Australia, and made a grim prediction: The earth's remaining indigenous societies, the experts warned, would see a dramatic decline in the course of this century. Whole bands and tribes could become wiped out, in some cases.

In the past, infectious diseases as well as the destruction and confiscation of the natural habitat led to the collapse of indigenous societies and cultures. Now, something new threatens the last remaining aborigines and islanders. The meeting in Melbourne was called Diabetes in Indigenous People Forum,[1] the first of its kind addressing the danger diabetes poses to these communities around the world.

Australia's aborigines and Torres Strait Islanders are just as much at risk as New Zealand's Maori and Native Americans in the United States and Canada. Small children in these communities, as young as six years old, have already fallen sick with type 2 diabetes. They are in danger of having heart attacks and failing kidneys later in life and are also at high risk of losing their eyesight.[2]

If you feel sorry for these indigenous peoples, however, you should not forget to feel sorry for your neighbors, acquaintances, friends, peers, relatives, and colleagues as well—and possibly for yourself. The fate of the Aborigines, Islanders, and Native Americans is our own fate, too. In terms of their genetic makeup, the members of all human ethnic groups are substantially identical. A sedentary New Yorker faces the same risks as a sedentary Navajo. And indeed, Western societies are in the middle of this crisis: Every ten seconds, a person somewhere in the industrialized world gets a limb amputated because of type 2 diabetes.

A GLOBAL EPIDEMIC

The epidemic of type 2 diabetes is a dire reminder that people today are genetically hardwired to pick berries and hunt mammoths. Two millions years ago, most hominids had a rather busy week. The men spent up to four days hunting; the women spent two to three days gathering food and other useful items. Physically demanding work was performed every day. Our forebears would carry their babies, kill and gut their prey, make stone tools, break bones open (to get the nutritious marrow), and build dwellings. Life was never boring and could change abruptly. In times when food was plentiful, people greedily devoured enormous portions of meat. During famine, however, they had so little food that they could starve to death.[3]

So, is modern civilization actually bad for us?

Of course not, and it doesn't require deep thinking to find reasons. Mean life expectancy is increasing every year by another three months, a trend that has endured for more than 160 years, chiefly driven by enhanced hygiene and safer food. Infant mortality is lower than ever. Heated houses, sanitary facilities, and health-care services have reduced the risk of death from infections and injuries, which were the most frequent causes of mortality 200 years ago.

And yet there are signs indicating that life expectancy, contrary to the predictions of many demographers, is about to level off and might even decline. "Looking out the window, we see a threatening storm—obesity—that will, if unchecked, have a negative effect on life expectancy," claims Jay Olshansky at the School of Public Health of the University of Illinois at Chicago, along with colleagues in an article in the *New England Journal of Medicine*.[4] Unless obesity among Americans is reduced, "the youth of today may, on average, live less healthy and possibly even shorter lives than their parents." A prognosis of the Department of Health in London arrives at a similarly grim prediction, stating that the mean life expectancy of Englishmen will be five years lower by the year 2050.

In the past, type 2 diabetes affected, if anyone, only people of old age. Today, the medical term "adult-onset diabetes" is outdated. One of every three children born in the United States in 2000 is going to suffer from type 2 diabetes at some point, often early in life. This will only add to the dramatic health disparities already existing in the United States. Women living in affluent neighborhoods of New Jersey have a mean life expectancy that is 30 years higher than that of women dwelling in parts of South Dakota.[5]

The gears of evolution grind slowly, making it impossible for our genetic makeup to adapt to the modern world. Today, the evolutionary program for energy conservation means that our muscle and bone tissues immediately begin to degrade as soon as we curl up on the sofa. If you don't use it, you will lose it. The resulting obesity and metabolic changes fuel the diabetes epidemic.

For some creatures, however, idle time does not always lead to a rapid degradation of bodily structures. Black bears, for example, rest five to seven months during the winter and retain most of their strength. Upon leaving their dens in the spring, the bears are in good shape and eager for activity. After 130 days of dormancy, the muscle strength of a bear's leg has declined by 23 percent, whereas a human leg would lose 90 percent of its power during the same period of rest. The difference lies in the genes. Black bears have evolved a metabolism suitable for hibernation. Certain biochemical mechanisms see to it that the bear's muscular system is not wasting away in the den.[6]

We humans are wired in a different way. We need exercise, much as we need air for breathing. We've inherited bodies that depend upon regular moderate activity. However, it is also the excess supply of food that does not agree with us. Humans evolved in times when famines abounded. Thus, after overeating, the body is not going to flush away all these superfluous sodas, sundaes, and pizzas. Instead, it converts all these calories into padding of sheer fat.

Curiously, humans are not the sole creatures unable to say "no" in front of a full plate. Cats and dogs also lack an instinct that would stop them from overeating. The masters and their pets are in the same boat: apparently 20 percent of all cats and dogs in the United States are obese. They, too, are at risk of getting cancer, type 2 diabetes, and arthritis. And American veterinarians have noticed another remarkable fact: the obese pets frequently resemble their mistresses and masters. "We see large numbers of domesticated pets being fed very high quality food and living very sedentary lifestyles with very limited exercise," says Scott Alan Brown at the University of Georgia in Athens. "Quite honestly, it's analogous to what we see in the pet owners."[7]

This excessive supply of sugar and fat has changed the constitution of a whole generation. This metamorphosis is especially evident when people gain access to unlimited food in a relatively short period of time. In West Germany, it happened shortly after the Second World War, when the first beer bellies popped up. Other researchers note the Pima Indians, a tribe whose people live in Mexico and the United States. Those in the United States consume 500 to 600 kilocalories a day more than their counterparts across the border. The result of this is that the Pima in the United States are on average 26 kilograms heavier and have one of the highest rates of type 2 diabetes in the world, some 50 percent of the population.

The onset of this metabolic disease is a textbook example of how much humans are still adapted to the Stone Age. The body is capable of storing only a small amount of sugar (glucose) in the liver and in the muscles. This supply becomes depleted after only one day of fasting. For this reason, the body needs a regulatory circuit protecting its glucose supply during a famine—which is why resting muscles are unable to fish glucose out of the bloodstream.

"Consequently, it would have been advantageous to our ancestors to develop a system that allowed only physically active muscles to remove blood glucose," explains Frank Booth at the University of Missouri in Columbia.[8] For the average American, who consumes fast food and drives everywhere, this ancient system now fires back. Underused muscles are not able to suck the glucose out of the bloodstream, and the blood then becomes thickened with sugar. This metabolic turmoil actually led to the name of the disease "diabetes mellitus" because those affected drink a lot of liquids and subsequently flush out unusually high amounts of urine (the term comes from the Greek *diabainein*, meaning "to flow through"). On the other hand, the urine contains high levels of sugar and is sweet; thus the term "mellitus" (derived from the Greek *meli*, or "honey").

In reaction to the excess amounts of glucose molecules in the blood, the body starts to produce high amounts of the hormone insulin. It is made in the pancreas and helps the muscle cells filter glucose out of the blood. The high levels of insulin, however, have unintended consequences: the cells stop responding to the abundant glucose molecules, instead becoming resistant. Subsequently, the whole glucose metabolism spins out of control, and the affected person falls sick with type 2 diabetes.

The disease progresses incrementally, and in the beginning there are no symptoms that can be felt, with the possible exception of fatigue and thirst. Furthermore, some affected men lose interest in sex. These sexual problems are caused by diabetic changes in the blood vessels and by the resulting impairment of the blood circulation in the pelvis, but patients erroneously blame their age for their loss of potency.

Before the Second World War, a person suffering from type 2 diabetes was a medical curiosity. Only 0.4 percent of the

German population suffered from adult-onset diabetes, as the condition was then known. Today, 10 percent of Germans are affected.[9] In the United States, the figures are also skyrocketing: according to the National Institutes of Health, approximately 19 to 20 million Americans have type 2 diabetes, and about one-third of them don't even know it. Diabetes prevalence in the United States has increased by 49 percent from 1990 to 2000 and is now believed to be the sixth leading cause of death in this country.[10]

Yet many patients regard type 2 diabetes as nothing but an annoying condition that could be easily managed and controlled. Ironically, medical advances have given rise to this popular fallacy. Canadian researchers discovered in 1921 that diabetes was caused by a lack of insulin. In the wake of this discovery, scientists found ways to produce insulin outside the human body that could be administered to patients. This treatment made it possible to keep even people in advanced stages of diabetes alive. Furthermore, pharmaceutical companies began producing so-called antidiabetic drugs. Although experts doubted the effectiveness of these products, their ready availability tricked patients into believing there was a quick fix for their problems. Additionally, manufacturers introduced expensive food products like diabetics' chocolate, pudding, and marmalade. This created the illusion among diabetic people that they could lead a more or less normal life, as long as they consumed the many products from pharmaceutical and food companies.

Patients' optimism, however, turned out to be premature. Many of the people who have simply rejected admonitions to exercise now have to face the dire consequences of their decisions. Even though people with type 2 diabetes can survive for a surprisingly long time, they don't have a particularly enjoyable life. The long-term consequences of the disease are severe. For one, the circulation becomes weak, and the kidneys often stop working, making dialysis necessary. The high level of glucose in the blood can destroy the retina, a fatal degeneration causing blindness. Eye damage is thought to occur in 19 percent of diabetics.

Moreover, the sugar in the blood attacks nerve cells in the feet and in the legs. Problems such as amputation of a toe or a foot, foot lesions, and numbness in the feet occur in 23 percent of people with diabetes. And sadly, an amputation usually further worsens the lack of exercise that promoted the onset of type 2 diabetes in the first place.

EXERCISE TO TREAT DIABETES

Proof that physical activity is effective in treating diabetes is the outcome of a whole array of studies. In the Chinese city of Daqing, sedentary persons who already showed early symptoms of the disease were allowed to keep their drinking and eating habits, but only if they committed themselves to regular exercise. Six years later their risk for developing full-blown type 2 diabetes was cut by 46 percent. Individuals in a control group conversely stayed sedentary but changed their eating habits. They only reduced their risk by 31 percent.[11]

In one trial, 3,234 overweight Americans at the onset of type 2 diabetes (they had impaired glucose tolerance) were randomly divided into three different groups. The members of the first group were given a daily dose of the standard medication: two tablets of metformin to slow down the glucose production in the liver, thereby lowering the level of glucose in the blood. The patients of the second group received placebo pills. The members of the third group were encouraged to change their lifestyle: They were asked to go on a low-fat diet and to walk for 30 minutes, five days a week, with the goal of losing 7 percent of their body weight.

After three years, all the participants of the study were re-examined. In the group taking the standard medication, the prevalence of the disease in comparison with the group receiving placebo was reduced by 31 percent. However, the individuals prescribed the walking treatment were in better health, with the prevalence of the condition lowered by 58 percent.[12]

Spanish physicians prescribed ten men with fully developed type 2 diabetes a moderate form of exercise. Over four months, the patients exercised two days per week, but did not have to change their eating habits (their intake of energy in the food actually rose by 15 percent). The result: The total average weight of the participants remained the same, but the fat distribution had shifted toward a more benign pattern. The fat deposits around the belly that are believed to be particularly bad for one's health shrank by 10 percent. Furthermore, the blood-sugar levels dramatically improved. These findings show that regular exercise pays off, even when it isn't accompanied by loss of weight.[13]

Statisticians at the University of Leicester in England wanted to know whether lifestyle changes could even turn around the symptoms of an emerging diabetic sickness. Recently, they carried out a survey of the medical literature and tracked down a total of 17 trials, covering 8,084 subjects. This meta-analysis revealed that "lifestyle interventions seem to be at least as effective as pharmacological interventions," with the additional bonus of creating fewer adverse reactions. The survey is good news for people already showing early symptoms of diabetes: moderate exercise can cut the risk of fully contracting this insidious illness by half.[14]

For healthy people, it's also worth heeding this advice because the onset of diabetes is inversely correlated to the fitness of a person. This is the central message of a large epidemiological study involving more than 84,000 nurses: If you eat a balanced diet, avoid becoming overweight, are a nonsmoker, drink modest amounts of alcohol, and exercise for 30 minutes a day, you will dramatically increase your chances of never getting diabetes in the first place.[15]

5

Muscles and Metabolism

A NUMBER OF YEARS AGO, 12 MEN GATHERED IN BOSTON BECAUSE they were fed up with having lost their physical strength. One of them was Arthur, a 62-year-old dockworker. During his whole career, Arthur was used to physical labor, until he was promoted to being a foreman at age 50. From then on, he usually had to carry responsibility rather than heavy weights. But some days, Arthur's muscle strength was needed to help carry boxes full of scrap iron. To the amusement of his underlings, Arthur was too feeble to lift them. Manuel, another member of the flabby dozen, had a similar experience. At age 70 he was delighted to be a grandfather, but he was too weak to lift his three-year-old granddaughter.

Arthur, Manuel, and the other ten men volunteered to participate in a unique experiment designed by the physician Irwin Rosenberg and his colleagues at the renowned Human Nutrition Research Center on Aging at Tufts University in Boston. The researchers wanted to test a formula against the symptoms of aging. "We were not focusing on the cosmetic aspects of aging, those visible signs of decline—sagging skin, age spots, receding hairlines, more pronounced facial features, and the like—that cause people so much anguish and create a huge market for beauty products companies," recounted Rosenberg, whom I met in his office at Tufts. Rather, he wanted to give back the men their lost vitality—an undertaking many considered impossible and dubious. Back then, many physicians, as well as a wide swath of the population, assumed withering away was a natural and inescapable part of getting old.

Irwin Rosenberg, however, was thinking outside the box. At one point it struck him that many older persons around him were leading strange lives. They didn't have major illnesses like cancer or heart disease, and yet they weren't living by themselves, instead depending on nursing assistance. These people were smart and in good shape mentally—but for some reason, their bodies were falling apart. Rosenberg had a hunch: In reality, these seniors had the full potential of being healthy. Their symptoms were not related to specific diseases but rather had been caused by the long period without physical activity and the resulting wasting away of muscle cells. These people were simply too weak to be healthy. In an effort to raise awareness of their plight, Rosenberg, as noted, proposed a new name: Sarcopenia, an overlooked phenomenon that, he suspected, should not be mistaken as a natural part of the aging process.

In order to prove his assumption, Rosenberg turned to the flabby dozen for help. To begin with, the 12 volunteers, aged 60 to 72, were thoroughly examined, then participated for three months in a training program three days a week. Arthur, Manuel, and the others were asked to do weight lifting at 80 percent of their maximum (defined as the heaviest weight a person can lift one time). Subsequently, they were examined again. Using lab tests, microscopic analysis, and magnetic resonance imaging, the doctors documented the changes after three months of training.

The results exceeded the expectations of physicians and participants alike. Arthur, the foreman, was able to triple his muscle strength. Initially, he could lift a weight of only 50 pounds, but now he could lift almost 150 pounds. Moreover, after the end of the study, he continued working out. As a consequence, his chronic back pain eventually disappeared. "From Arthur's point of view, the best bonus of all was being able to keep up with the younger guys at the loading dock, much to their amazement and his amusement," Rosenberg recounts.[1]

Similarly, Manuel, the proud but weak grandfather, felt like a new man. Over the course of the study, the size of his leg muscles increased by 17 percent, and he lost more than 13 pounds of fat. The average result of the dozen participants was truly encouraging. Their muscle strength increased two to three times over, and their muscle mass grew by 10 to 15 percent.

NEVER TOO LATE

Shortly after this remarkable study, the young doctor Maria Fiatarone (now Maria Fiatarone Singh) joined the team at Tufts. She proposed a new study, the results of which became a milestone in sports medicine. Fiatarone went to the Hebrew Rehabilitation Center for the Aged, in Boston, and encouraged ten women and men aged 87 to 96 to train for eight weeks. Despite their advanced age, these courageous women and men were asked to train at 80 percent of their maximum capacity. The result of this test was greeted with awe: The mass of their thigh muscles grew by more than 10 percent, and their muscle strength almost tripled.

To Fiatarone, the most critical question was whether these changes actually improved the lives of her ten senior test subjects. Thus she asked them to walk a 20-foot course and found that the training indeed translated into increased quickness and sureness of step. These results also enhanced the mental mood of the elderly participants. "Every day I feel better, more optimistic," said Sam Semansky, aged 93, who could get around again without a walker. "Pills won't do for you what exercise does!"[2]

Fiatarone continued her career and went on to hold the John Sutton Chair of Exercise and Sport Science at the University of Sydney. Irwin Rosenberg remained in Boston and watched his predictions proven right by many other studies. We actually can get back our vitality. True, no one can defy death. But we can systematically increase the number of healthy days in our lives. "We age biologically, not chronologically," says Rosenberg. "If you maintain function, you can overcome the biological process." Even individuals who have not jumped rope or have not run after a ball in years can have a second chance. Advanced age is "a dynamic state that, in most people, can be changed for the better no matter how many years they've lived or neglected their body in the past."[3]

ACTIVATING GENES

This chance for renewal is due to the amazing plasticity of our muscle system. There are more than 600 different muscles in the body, and the skeletal muscles (they execute our deliberate motions) comprise a huge organ that together account for about 50 percent of the body weight in a lean individual. Until recently, sports doctors were mainly interested in the heart, but now their attention is shifting toward these muscles and the larger study of the biology that makes us fit.[4]

Muscle cells can be changed rather easily. They always respond to motion and strain: The size, strength, and contraction speed of single fibers depends on stimulation. Physical exercise affects the nucleus of a muscle cell and influences the production of certain genes and proteins. Molecular biologists are starting to study these processes and hope to gain insights allowing the development of better training methods.

Researchers have also discovered that our muscles play a key role in our health. Strengthening muscles changes their physiological composition, which, in turn, benefits other processes in the body. And now, scientists are finally beginning to understand the mechanics of muscle wasting. As we saw in chapter 2, after only a few days of rest, our muscles shrink. Contrary to popular belief, this atrophy is not a passive side effect of laziness but an active cellular process under the control of a specific set of genes. Inside the cell, some muscle proteins are chemically marked, allowing digestive enzymes to detect and chop them into amino acids, which are then used for other purposes. In the process, the fibers inside the cells are incrementally degraded, and the cells themselves get thinner and weaker—although they remain alive.

Apparently at least 90 different genes control such atrophy, the so-called atrogenes. The atrogenes are thought to be a legacy of our Stone Age past. Our odds of survival increase when we do not have to invest energy to maintain muscles that are simply idle.

Conversely, other genetic circuits control the buildup of new muscle structures. One part of the circuit was discovered when a remarkable boy was born in Berlin in 1999. He came into the world with a fully developed musculature, and by age four was allegedly so strong that he could hold a weight of more than six pounds with his extended arm. The pediatrician Markus Schülke, at Charité University Hospital in Berlin, discovered that this boy had a rare genetic mutation and lacked a protein, myostatin, that usually limits the growth of muscle cells. Additional tests revealed the boy's mother had a very similar mutation and possessed only minute levels of myostatin. Small wonder she was a very successful sprinter in her younger years.[5]

Under normal circumstances, the growth of certain muscles is triggered and controlled by bodily motions. In experiments, animals that are kept for four months in an environment where they can run every day on a treadmill will double the amount of small blood vessels in their muscles, as well as the number of mitochondria, the power plants of the cell. Obviously, muscle cells are able to sense physical demands and respond accordingly.

The physiologist Darrell Neufer, at John B. Pierce Laboratory in New Haven, Connecticut, has studied how this sensing system might work. In one test, he and his colleagues encouraged volunteers to repeat an exercise for 90 minutes on five consecutive days. They used only one leg to lift a weight that was 70 percent of their maximum capacity. On the fifth day, the researchers performed biopsies on both legs, removing tiny bits of muscle tissue from the trained and untrained limbs. The biopsies were carried out at different times: before training, immediately afterward, and many hours after. Finally, the researchers analyzed which kinds of genes had been activated in the muscle samples.[6]

As expected, exercise had turned on a wide array of genes playing key roles in the metabolism. But surprisingly, this gene activity did not peak during or immediately after exercise. Rather, there was a time lag. Two to four hours after the workout, as the leg was recovering, the gene activity reached its maximum. It is this delayed response that allows the muscle to adapt to physical strain. Hours after exercise, new proteins are produced so that the muscle can grow. After a while, however, these proteins become degraded, which explains why repetition is so important. Only if the exercise is performed regularly will the level of proteins remain high. This cumulative effect finally makes us fit.

The composition of muscle cells is equally important because skeletal muscle cells can be subdivided into distinct types. At one end of the spectrum is type-II-b. These are known as fast-twitch glycolytic muscles. They can act quickly because they burn up glycogen. They are quite strong but quickly get fatigued. They contain only a few mitochondria (about 1 percent of the cellular volume).

At the other end of the spectrum is type-I. These slow-twitch oxidative muscles chiefly oxidize fatty acids as fuel. They are not terribly strong but have endurance and contain many mitochondria (3 to 10 percent of the cellular volume). In addition, there are more subtypes such as fast-twitch oxidative, also containing abundant mitochondria.

While the classification of all these subtypes might appear confusing, they have a profound influence on our health. The more oxidative muscles we have, the better. Most persons actually have a mosaic of the different subtypes. The pattern is first set over the course of the embryonic development and can greatly vary among individuals. The proportion of desirable type-I muscles ranges from 13 to 96 percent and averages 50 to 60 percent. Individuals bearing many type-I muscles are often good endurance runners.[7]

TRANSFORMING THE BODY

Until recently it was assumed that we cannot control our muscle-type patterns. But the physiologists Jan Carlsson and Bengt Saltin started to study the molecular details and soon abandoned the old tenet. In animal experiments, for example, it has been shown that individuals can alter whole muscles, from one type to the other, and back again. The physician R. Sanders Williams, at Duke University Medical Center in Durham, North Carolina, says, "Whatever the genetic predisposition is—the effect of physical activity is predominant."[8]

Each healthy human, fat or lean, is able to change the composition of his or her muscles by using them. If muscle cells are idle most of the time and are only occasionally used for heavy tasks, they morph into type-II-b and are not particularly good for our well-being.

However, jogging and bicycle riding stimulate muscle cells and turn them into the much-preferred oxidative muscles with their widespread benefits. Beyond bestowing endurance and stamina on our bodies, they will benefit the body's metabolism.

We can exploit this throughout life because our astonishing muscular plasticity remains intact even in old age. As Williams states: "You don't need stem cells to be fit." Rather, you can use regular exercise to outfit and supply your body systematically with healthful oxidative muscles.

Exercise not only changes the composition of the muscular system but also a whole range of measurements throughout the body. Irwin Rosenberg has come up with ten distinct measurements he calls "biomarkers."[9] By following these biomarkers during a training period, one can show that exercise invariably helps the body. The growth of the muscle mass and the increase of strength, two of the biomarkers, are effects one would expect above all. But Rosenberg and his colleagues at Tufts University have identified others as well.

Basal Metabolic Rate

The term metabolism refers to the many biochemical processes occurring constantly in our body. The basal metabolic rate describes the total sum of these processes while the body is resting, whether in the morning, when we sleepily open our eyes, or at night, when we nod off. Over the course of time our basal metabolic rate incrementally decreases. Thus a 25-year-old woman sleeping burns more calories than her 80-year-old grandmother, who weighs the same and is also having a siesta.

For many years, researchers had a hard time identifying the causes of this age-related decline of the basal metabolic rate. After a lot of guesswork, they discovered how body composition plays a crucial role. When a person has a small muscle mass—as is typically the case with middle-aged people who have neglected to exercise for many years—then the metabolism needs less oxygen and energy; fat tissue requires less fuel than muscle tissue.

This difference points to two ways to avoid gaining weight over time. One can cut back consumption of calories by exactly the amount the metabolic rate sinks, which would amount to 100 fewer kilocalories per day for every decade of life after age 20. The second option would be to get moving and increase one's basal metabolic rate.

Relative Body Fat

Even when people are not adding weight while aging, their body fat usually increases. Rosenberg and colleagues examined hundreds of elderly people and quantified this tendency: The average 65-year-old sedentary woman consists of 43 percent body fat, whereas a 25-year-old woman typically has 25 percent fat. For men, things are similar: 65-year-olds average 38 percent fat, whereas 25-year-old men average 18 percent.

For older people to achieve a more youthful ration, other than eating less, they have to remain physically active. If they walked every day for two kilometers, they would burn 140 kilocalories respectively each day. After one year, that would be 51,000 kilocalories, and nearly 18 pounds of fat tissue would have melted away.[10]

Aerobic Capacity

To keep living, to refresh our blood, humans must breathe oxygen. Aerobic capacity measures the consumption of oxygen in a given time. Compared to young adults, people at age 65 have an aerobic capacity that is 30 to 40 percent lower.

Once again, we can slow down this decline with physical exercise. Aerobic capacity indicates our fitness level. Moreover, muscle type also influences it. The healthful oxidizing muscle type virtually sucks oxygen out of the bloodstream. Thus if you are elevating your aerobic capacity by physical activity, it is a sure sign that you have increased the percentage of desirable oxidizing muscle types.

Blood Sugar Tolerance

This describes the body's ability to control the amount of glucose in the blood, thereby avoiding the damaging effects seen in diabetic individuals. Strength training and physical exercise increase muscle mass, which (by way of insulin signals) can soak up glucose. On balance, this improves the blood sugar tolerance.

Bone Density

Bones grow when they are used. The bigger the effort, the stronger they get. A study from Finland revealed that professional squash players have bone densities 15 percent higher in the arm they play with compared to nonplayers. Physical activity boosts the incorporation of calcium ions into bones, making these more robust and sturdier. The rate of this incorporation is directly correlated to the number of years training.[11]

Internal Temperature

"Our bodies come with a built-in thermostat," says Rosenberg.[12] Whether it is humid or chilly in our environment, the body is always able to keep its working temperature of about 98 degrees Fahrenheit. Sweating cools us down, while shivering warms us up. This control system is closely related to the aerobic capacity and the balance of electrolytes in the body, which in turn can be positively influenced by exercise.

Cholesterol: Amount and Type

Our bodies cannot function without cholesterol, and they are even capable of producing it when cholesterol is absent from food. The human brain consists of 10 to 20 percent cholesterol (based on the dry mass), and depends on a steady supply. Because the substance is too fatty to circulate by itself through the bloodstream, certain proteins, called lipoproteins, must transport it. However, when the concentration of certain lipoproteins is highly elevated, it creates a risk of cardiovascular diseases.[13]

William E. Kraus at the Duke University Medical Center has found that a certain type of exercise is especially good at keeping lipoproteins in check: longer spells of moderate exercise seem to be more beneficial than shorter, more intensive workouts. Jogging 12 miles per week reduces the number of small, unwanted lipoproteins, but jogging for 20 miles per week produces even better results.[14]

Blood Pressure

The pressure inside the blood vessels and the lungs is determined by the capacity of the heart, viscosity of the blood, and the resistance created by the blood vessels. Researchers have demonstrated in more than 50 trials that regular endurance training lowers blood pressure, and that even rather modest everyday activities translate into measurable improvements. Exercise is thus a proven and reliable remedy for people with hypertension, although this is not widely appreciated. For one thing, many people with high blood pressure lack motivation to work out. But frequently the treating doctors are to blame, says Hans-Georg Predel of the Sports University in Cologne, Germany. He has made the sobering observation that physicians "often don't consider the effectiveness of an intervention without drugs and that they lack a sufficient expertise in prescribing lifestyle changes."[15]

Biological Age

The sports physicians at Tufts were among the first to demonstrate that all of these biomarkers will improve when an out-of-shape person starts to exercise.[16] They came up with a mix of light endurance (brisk walking and bicycling) and modest strength exercises that can be easily done at home. Time and again, researchers found that anyone who really follows the program for 16 weeks will reap the benefit of many improved bodily functions. It is important not to focus on these biomarkers as risk factors but rather as motivating numbers used to document gains.

What if you didn't know your age? That's a question Irwin Rosenberg asks. He tells the story of Satchel Paige, the legendary twentieth-century baseball player. Paige grew up poor in Alabama, and his parents had not noted his date of birth. Later in life, the pitcher used to say folks should guess his age by judging his performance in the ballpark. According to this measurement, Paige hardly aged at all because his outstanding career lasted for three decades.

Where Paige had his scores to show off, we have the biomarkers that reveal our true age. If you don't like the verdict of the biomarkers, you can change it. Just get moving.

6

What the Heart Desires

Fifty years ago, people who survived a heart attack were prescribed up to six months of bed rest. Walking and running, the doctors feared, would only trigger more infarctions, damaged areas of the heart. This mind-set was prevalent when President Dwight Eisenhower suffered a heart attack in 1955. A cardiologist named Paul Dudley White treated the ailing president.

White and Eisenhower were convinced the president would overcome his condition and live a long life. But many other doctors and wide segments of the American population were skeptical, especially after learning about the procedures White advocated. The doctor turned out to be an unusual fitness devotee who rode his bicycle to work and considered bed rest for patients to be nonsense. Instead, White prescribed his presidential patient doses of physical activity. Before long, sensational photographs were printed in newspapers showing heart patient Eisenhower playing golf. But White had done the right thing: Eisenhower recovered and, after being re-elected, was able to serve a second term.

Since then, physical activity has been considered a reliable remedy to slow down, halt, and even reverse heart disease, as well as a prophylactic that keeps a healthy heart young and resilient. Walking and training regularly decreases the risk of heart disease by 35 to 37 percent. Quitting smoking, shedding body fat, and switching to a balanced diet can dramatically enhance this effect, lowering the risk for coronary disease by 83 percent.[1]

In many trials, researchers have assessed the relationship between physical fitness and life expectancy. The lower the fitness level, the shorter the life, on average. Being out of shape is, according to these studies, as dangerous as smoking cigarettes. However, poor fitness is not a death warrant. In one study, sedentary people were retested after five years. Those who had started to exercise were rewarded for their lifestyle changes, with a mortality rate declining by 44 percent.[2]

SPORTS AS MEDICATION FOR THE HEART

Heart disease occurs when the small vessels in the heart muscle, the coronaries, are not sufficiently supplied with blood, a condition typically caused by arteriosclerosis. If the blood supply is interrupted for more than 20 minutes, the cells in the affected area will start to die—an infarction, which can be fatal. In sum, nearly half of the deaths in the United States and other industrialized countries are caused by cardiovascular disease.

In the fight against this killer, physical exercise has been found to trigger physiological changes that mirror the pharmacological effects of standard drugs. Consequently, in Germany, men and women suffering from heart disease train together in more than 6,000 sports groups supervised by physicians and professional personnel.[3] The participants benefit greatly, as revealed in a survey including 48 trials, with 8,940 patients: regular exercise reduced mortality attributable to heart disease by 26 percent.

In addition, physically active heart patients have significantly fewer heart attacks, fewer bypass operations, and fewer angioplasty procedures for widening atherosclerotic arteries. In effectiveness, physical exercise compares to established drugs like ACE-inhibitors (given after an infarction), but without adverse side effects.[4]

Although sudden physical exhaustion, especially when occurring after years of inactivity, might increase the risk of heart attacks and strokes, regular aerobic training is beneficial for thinning the blood. Moderate training not only improves cholesterol levels, blood pressure, and glucose tolerance, but also has a beneficial impact on the viscosity of the blood and reduces its tendency to form dangerous clots.

Exercise also helps individuals suffering from narrowed arteries and impaired circulation in the legs. Patients with this problem find that walking causes terrible aches in their legs, known as ischemic pain, forcing them to rest frequently. Yet using these legs helps to cure this disease because regular walking incrementally improves the endurance of the legs. In clinical studies, exercise helped increase the maximum distance a patient could walk without feeling ischemic pain by 179 percent, while the maximum distance a person could walk at all went up by 122 percent.[5]

In a survey comparing walking to angioplasty, the common treatment of dilating and sometimes placing a stent in

the affected vessels, angioplasty seemed slightly more effective than walking. But angioplasty can cause severe side effects. Another trial examined whether open-heart surgery is
superior to exercise. The result was that both treatments
were equally effective, but surgical interventions gave rise to
complications in 18 percent of the cases. In the case of
blood-thinning pills, exercise came out well ahead. Taking
such drugs increased the period of pain-free walking by 38
percent, but patients who simply exercised more improved
by 86 percent.[6]

OPENING UP BLOOD VESSELS

In looking at biological rather than chronological age, one can
say that we are as old as our arteries. The health of arteries is
a complex matter in which the inner lining of the blood vessels, the endothelium, plays a key role. This thin layer of cells
controls the muscle tone of the vessels. A malfunction of the
endothelium is one of the first symptoms of the onset of arteriosclerosis, as plaques build up inside the vessels.

In one remarkable trial published in the *New England Journal of Medicine*, individuals with heart disease trained on stationary bikes, for ten minutes at a time, six times per day—and
significantly improved their endothelium function and thus
the blood supply to the heart. The study showed that physical
activity can reverse the initial hardening of the arteries.[7]

Even when arteriosclerosis has progressed significantly, as is
often the case with older people, exercise is a felicitous remedy. The American researcher Dean Ornish became famous

after finding that regular exercise and a low-fat diet can widen narrowed vessels by approximately 5 percent.

Since then, researchers at the University of Göttingen, Germany, have confirmed that exercise does cause favorable changes in the condition of blood vessels. They experimented with mice genetically engineered to suffer from arteriosclerosis. Some mice were kept sedentary as controls, others were active. After running on treadmills five days per week for one hour, over a three-week span, the mice were deliberately injured at the left carotid artery, then put back on the treadmill program for three more weeks. Finally these mice were thoroughly examined. In comparison with the sedentary mice in the control group, the active runners had fewer atherosclerotic plaques and fewer constricted arteries. Furthermore, their wounds had healed better because connective tissue cells had grown to stabilize them.[8] Although physical exercise cannot completely prevent the slow progression of arteriosclerosis with age, these results show that it can significantly reduce the problems the disease may cause.

NEW ARTERIES FROM STEM CELLS

One of the most dramatic effects of exercise on the body is to promote the growth of new cells and blood vessels. That was shown in a human trial that involved exercising for eight weeks. New vessels, so-called collateral vessels, established new paths of circulation. This could mean that by getting moderate exercise, you are able to grow natural bypasses in your heart.[9]

In the past, most researchers thought the growth of collateral circulation was initiated by branches of the vessels that had been dormant or by vessels growing from neighboring areas into the area with the damage. But now they think an even more exciting mechanism is at work: Stem cells from the bone marrow are apparently capable of traveling specifically to blocked areas, where they morph into endothelial cells and start building new vessels.

Two studies performed at the University Hospital in Leipzig, Germany, have shown for the first time that these beneficial stem cells are multiplied by physical training. The hospital combines sports medicine with cardiology and employs not only doctors but also molecular biologists and one researcher with a degree in physical education. Their patients get exercise treadmills and stationary bikes, and their hearts are examined with ultrasound machines.

In one trial, researchers wanted to find out how the sick human heart is affected when patients train on stationary bikes.[10] The patients were asked to exercise until their chests started to ache; the pain signaled that the atherosclerotic heart muscle did not get enough oxygen. Two days after this test, the doctors took six blood samples and analyzed them in the laboratory. The results were startling: this *one* dose of exercise had caused a considerable release of stem cells from the bone marrow.

In another study, the physicians prescribed exercise for 18 men who had gotten themselves into lamentable physical shape.[11] They were sedentary and chain-smoking to the point of developing peripheral vascular disease, a lack of circulation, in their legs. On the treadmill, these men could not go faster than 2.2 miles per hour. Many of the patients stopped after walking only 50 to 200 meters because they experienced terrible leg aches.

This beneficial—if torturous—program lasted one month. Five days per week, the patients had to walk six times until they felt pain. In the course of their workouts, astonishing things happened inside their bodies. The number of stem cells in the blood tripled, and these cells apparently initiated the renewal of the malfunctioning vessel system for those with peripheral vascular disease in the legs. The investigating cardiologist, Rainer Hambrecht, believes his research tapped into a natural repair mechanism: "The body helps itself and tries, by releasing stem cells from the bone marrow, to promote the growth of new collateral circulation."[12]

According to these studies, heart patients do not have to train through the pain threshold to reap these beneficial effects. Whereas moderate training did not immediately cause the release of stem cells, more of them appeared in the blood after three months. Moreover, preexisting stem cells became activated, which "may in fact decelerate disease progression," as the researchers conclude in the journal *Circulation*.[13]

How do these effects compare to those achieved by fiddling with the symptoms of arteriosclerosis by using high-tech medicine? This was the subject of yet another landmark study from the center in Leipzig, of 100 men whose coronary arteries had already narrowed.[14] Half the patients were treated with angioplasty, the mechanical widening of narrowed or obstructed blood vessels, followed by the insertion of a mesh tube (or stent) to prop open an artery. The other half received a prescription called exercise: every day, these patients trained

As with heart failure, physical activity can help to overcome the problems caused by such illnesses as asthma and chronic bronchitis. Asthma is a chronic inflammatory irritation of the air passages that hampers the lungs through recurring attacks. Triggered by allergies as well as physical strain in cold weather, the bronchial tubes can suddenly narrow and start secreting mucus that blocks them. When this happens, a person can still breathe in, but can hardly breathe out, which leads to the frightening symptoms, like fierce coughing and shortness of breath.

Children with asthma are often excluded from physical education and sports and are encouraged to take it easy, which actually makes their troubles worse: Muscles waste away, which makes the children even less able to breathe properly, starting a vicious cycle.

Regular modest exercise would instead improve their bodies' resilience. Although the illness is not cured, people with asthma can become better at increasing the threshold for attacks, thereby avoiding them. Before starting, people with asthma should consult a specialist to work out an individual training plan.

for 20 minutes on a stationary bike at 70 percent of their maximum capacity.

After one year, the researchers compared the respective outcomes. Eighty-eight percent of the exercising patients avoided clinical events like additional angioplasty or even heart attacks. This was true for only 70 percent of the other patients. Many members of the stent group also needed the insertion of additional stents and on average had to be readmitted more often to the hospital because of recurring chest pain. The gentle exercise regimen, by comparison, was not only more effective but cheaper. On average, the treatment of one active patient necessitated medical costs of $3,429, whereas the average sedentary patient created $6,956 in costs.[15]

FRESH POWER FOR EXHAUSTED HEARTS

Those who spend time with patients suffering from heart failure might well feel that these patients should have their peace. After tiny bits of exercise, they gasp for breath, they get tired, and their legs become swollen. The underlying condition, cardiac insufficiency, can be caused by infections of the heart muscle, valve defects, and coronary arteriosclerosis. Until the 1970s, the standard treatment was strict bed rest. Too much strain, doctors believed, would further impair the heart, resulting in shortness of breath and swollen legs even at rest.

Today, doctors say the opposite is true. The paradigm began to shift when physicians realized that there is no direct causal connection between heart failure and general physical resilience. Instead, the problem lies with the skeletal muscles; those affected have atrophied muscles and are extremely feeble. Rather than letting their muscles waste away further, they should retrain their bodies.[16]

This new understanding of the disease led to studies showing that physical activity turns out to be an excellent remedy against heart failure. More than 25 trials have demonstrated that regular exercise improves the pulse rate, increases the maximum oxygen uptake, and decreases blood pressure. Most participants of these studies also took drugs to prevent heart failure, but the training brought additional benefits, namely an increase of 15 to 20 percent in the amount of exercise they could endure. Often this was critical in making the life of a sick person worth living again.

Heart patients who are not too excited about jogging might consider dancing. Italian researchers invited patients with heart failure to a dancing course that lasted eight weeks. These ladies and gentlemen gathered three days per week in the gym of the local hospital and danced for about 20 minutes. The dancers improved their physical condition to the same extent as volunteer patients in a control group who had trained on stationary bikes and treadmills. Not surprisingly, the dancers were much more motivated than the control-group patients, with more chances to laugh and maybe even flirt a little bit than those stuck on bikes or treadmills.[17]

Moderate exercise can also bring about changes at the molecular level. Doctors at the heart center of the University Hospital in Leipzig encouraged 12 patients with heart disease to exercise for six months: 20 minutes on the stationary bike every day, plus an hour walking or playing ball games every week. Subsequently, the researchers took samples from the flexor muscles of the patients' thighs.

The remarkable result, published in the journal *Circulation*, showed that the activity of so-called scavenger enzymes significantly increased in the muscles of the active patients, compared to 11 sedentary individuals with heart disease. These enzymes are beneficial because they remove aggressive substances known as free radicals, which can harm the heart muscle.[18]

Unfortunately, these discoveries have not yet reached all patients and physicians. Even half a century after the miraculous recovery of President Eisenhower, the healing power of exercise is withheld from many individuals with heart disease. Despite all the clear-cut advantages and benefits, states the cardiologist Paul D. Thompson of Hartford Hospital, "exercise training is rarely prescribed for cardiac patients, as evidenced by the fact that only about 20 percent of qualified patients are referred to formal cardiac rehabilitation programs. Among women and older patients referral rates are even lower."[19]

7

Growing Bones

WHEN THE JOINTS HURT AND THE BONES ACHE, MOST PEOPLE would rather stay in bed. But as with other problems we've discussed, this will only lead to more trouble. Perhaps lying down might spare the cartilage, that smooth and elastic lining of the joints that makes sure bones do not grind painfully on each other when used. Yet it is not only the cartilage that helps your joints. The surrounding muscles also guard and protect joints because they cushion the jolts that damage a moving body. Thanks to muscles, cartilage absorbs fewer shocks.

For that reason, physical inactivity is like poison for the joints. The more muscles waste away, the more bumps and jolts directly affect the cartilage, gradually wearing it down. This way, bones start to ache, people become less active, muscles shrink more, and cartilage gets battered even harder—not a happy trend. A joint may end up being completely destroyed so that it must be replaced with an artificial one. Or the threat looms of being moved to a retirement home. Neither dementia nor problems caused by arteriosclerosis are the most frequent reason for being institutionalized; most people are admitted because they suffer from an ailing musculoskeletal system.

But there's hope. People can't reclaim lost cartilage, but they can definitely increase muscle mass. In this way, you can renew the guardians of your joints, preventing future disease, and cure existing ailments.[1]

STRENGTHENING RATHER THAN REPLACING JOINTS

At about 120 different spots in the body, two bones are connected with joints. Unfortunately, not all of them are perfect links. The term *arthritis* covers more than 100 distinct conditions relating to joint problems, and each one can make life miserable. There are two types of arthritis: inflammatory and degenerative. Common osteoarthritis belongs to the latter one; mechanical forces drive the destruction of cartilage, mainly of the knee and the hip. Among 34-year-old people, about 17 percent suffer from osteoarthritis; among people of age 65 or older, the figure is more than 90 percent. Once the cartilage is gone, the disease can progress rapidly, resulting in bulky joints, thickened bones, muscular atrophy, and inflammations that ravage the capsules that cushion the joints.

People notice this degeneration because of the pain developing over time. Initially, the pain occurs only when the affected joints are moved or touched. After a while, the aches become chronic, and the joints swell. At this point, many patients unconsciously cut down on physical activity—and unwittingly worsen their ailments.

Severely arthritic knees have become a huge and lucrative field within the medical industry: Patients are either instructed to take expensive drugs or to get artificial joints implanted. Yet the researcher Miriam Nelson, at Tufts University in Boston, seems to be convinced there is another way: The best remedy may be for stricken patients to help themselves by strengthening the affected leg muscles.

Nelson and her colleagues have developed a 16-week training program that can be done at home with a stool and light ankle weights.[2] The researchers tested their program with 46 volunteers who were in virtually constant pain and were hardly able to walk or climb stairs. The researcher Kristin Baker, part of the Tufts team, visited the patients at home and told half of them how to do the exercises. The other patients also received house calls, but during these visits, Baker just talked in broad terms about the disease and tried to lift the patients' spirits a little.

Subsequently, the researchers compared the outcomes of the two groups. The patients of the training group reported they had significantly less pain and could perform 17 different physical tasks much better than the inactive patients. The average pain level of the exercising group had plummeted by 43 percent, compared to 12 percent for the inactive patients. The physical performance of the first group improved by 44 percent, nearly twice as much as in the placebo group, which the researchers attribute to muscular resilience; the strength of the thigh muscles increased by 71 percent.

"All of a sudden, people who had founds life's daily activities more and more challenging and painful as a result of arthritis pain were able to participate in life in ways they hadn't been able to for years," states Miriam Nelson. "The exercisers were able to walk, climb stairs, sit, and stand more easily. And they slept more easily."[3]

By now, these landmark findings have been confirmed many times. A large survey of 786 patients with worn-out knee joints has also shown that people who exercise the muscles surrounding their affected knee are rewarded with significantly less pain. In order to reap this benefit, it was necessary to work out only 20 to 30 minutes per day with elastic straps.[4]

The training does more than reduce pain. People adopting an exercise regimen can use their joints much better than before. In a trial of 250 patients aged 60 or older, the participants had chronic pain but were still mobile. They could get up without support, went to the bathroom alone, and dressed themselves. In the study, they were randomly assigned to three different groups. The members of the first one were asked to walk briskly three days per week. After three months, the first part of the program ended, but the volunteers were encouraged to keep their newly acquired walking habit.

The members of the second group were instructed to do nine different exercises at a weight-lifting machine. They, too, were asked to continue after the initial three-month period. Finally, there was a control group who received general information about osteoarthritis but were not prescribed any exercise.

One year later, all participants were examined to see whether they could still keep up with the activities of daily life. The result: In the control group, 53 percent of the people had lost the ability to live without assistance. In the other two groups, that was true only for 37 percent, no matter what type of activity they did. The more diligently a person trained, the better the result. Overall, the success rate could have been even larger had all the volunteers lived up to their resolutions. But after 10 months, only 54 percent of them continued the exercises. The dropouts altered the outcome of the study and, worse, their own health.[5]

A review of the literature on osteoarthritic knees and exercise suggests that the type of exercise is less important than being active in the first place. Even moderate activities, like doing the Chinese martial art tai chi three days per week, bring promising results, Jean-Michel Brismée and colleagues at the Texas Tech University Health Sciences Center, in Lubbock, Texas, have found.[6] In those cases, patients' pain was relieved after only nine weeks, and the mobility of their joints improved. A recent study in the prestigious *New England Journal of Medicine* showed that arthroscopic surgery for osteoarthritis of the knee "provides no additional benefit to optimized physical and medical therapy."[7]

The results are remarkable, given that mainstream medicine strongly favors more aggressive therapy options like drugs or surgical procedures. About 300,000 knee replacement operations and more than 193,000 hip replacement surgeries are performed each year in the United States.[8] Even though these interventions are often necessary and a painkilling godsend for some patients, experts question whether so many are justified. "If we look at the age and objective discomforts of many patients who were advised to get an artificial hip, we cannot resist the impression that this operation was suggested very prematurely—long before the treatment with pills and other means like exercise and physiotherapy would have hit the wall," says the physician Klaus-Michael Braumann at Hamburg University, Germany.[9]

There are continuing concerns about the high rate of surgical joint replacement in Germany and in the United States because in both countries these interventions are costly for patients and insurers, and lucrative for doctors and hospitals.

RUNNING WITHOUT REMORSE

Another dangerous myth that keeps people sedentary is that running leads to the premature degradation of knee cartilage. Yet an increasing number of published medical articles indicate the opposite. According to these findings, all these women and men jogging through Central Park in Manhattan or along the Charles River in Boston are not ruining their knees. Actually, it is the large number of sedentary and often obese Americans who sit and lie around whose cartilage is more likely to be in decay.

However, it is very important which type of exercise one chooses. Soccer and downhill skiing are certainly not very good for knees. This is not because of the exercise as such, but because of the high risk of injury to key parts of the knee, such as the capsules under the kneecap, the kneecap itself, and the key ligament in the knee known as the cruciate ligament. Playing competitive sports does indeed increase the likelihood of suffering from osteoarthritis rather early in life. In one survey, doctors examined the knees of 117 men who formerly were elite athletes and found a lot of injuries: 14 percent of the examined soccer players had osteoarthritis, as did 31 percent of weight lifters.

But running is not among the sports with a high risk for getting injured. According to a study of 27 long-distance runners, the human body is capable of running 20 to 40 kilometers per week for 40 years without damage. Compared to 27 non-runners, these endurance athletes did not show any arthritic signs at the joints of hip, knee, and ankle.[10] A similar result was found among runners with an average age of 63 who were monitored for five years, again with no sign of increased cartilage loss.[11]

By contrast, inactive and obese people have a higher incidence of osteoarthritis, and there seems to be a direct correlation. More than 45 percent of patients with severely osteoarthritic knees carry around above-average weight. Obesity triggers the problem. At first a person becomes fat, then subsequently develops ailing knees. The same connection was found for the hip. Being overweight at age 40 significantly increases the risk for developing osteoarthritis of the hip.

We set our course in middle age, around 40. People who stop exercising by this age in order to protect their bones may actually cause the opposite effect. Jogging helps to reduce weight, which then relieves the joints.[12] Arthritis patients who are extremely overweight should be a little cautious, however. Instead of running, they should start out with bicycling and walking.

BEING RESTLESS, FIGHTING RHEUMATISM

While osteoarthritis is triggered by physical abrasion, so-called rheumatoid arthritis is a chronic inflammatory disease that at first usually affects one particular joint or a few of them. By the time patients see a doctor, about 50 percent of them are no longer able to use their wrists normally. Within the first two years of the disease, big joints usually become affected, and many patients experience severe symptoms. Pain, swelling, and stiffness make it extremely difficult for them to be physically active. This leads to predictable consequences; people with arthritis frequently lose muscle mass and are 30 to 70 percent weaker than healthy people. Their heart and lungs function worse, and their endurance is reduced by 50 percent.

Physiotherapy under supervision was for a long time the only physical activity that doctors allowed people with rheumatism. These cautious exercises helped the mobility of arthritis sufferers but not their fitness. For this purpose, aerobic training would have been needed—but physicians were reluctant to prescribe it to their patients because they were afraid it might bring even more damage to inflamed joints. However, it is turning out that this fear was unfounded. Many studies have shown that aerobic as well as strength training soothes the pain from rheumatism without showing any "increased disease activity or additional destruction of the joints," says the orthopedic specialist Stefan Gödde at the University Hospital of Saarland in Hamburg.[13] Most of the trials included patients with mild to severe symptoms.

Dutch researchers followed 300 patients with arthritis over the course of two years. One group of the participants received the standard treatment, whereas another group was prescribed exercise for two days per week: 20 minutes' training on a stationary bike; 20 minutes' strength training; and 20 minutes of games like soccer, badminton, basketball, and volleyball. The patients were reexamined every six months. Not only had their rheumatism not worsened, inflammatory processes in the joints were apparently soothed. Loss of bone density had slowed down, and overall fitness had improved, which in turn made the patients happier and more satisfied with their mental well-being.

FITNESS FOR FIBROMYALGIA

Fibromyalgia is still a medical mystery. Although some physicians doubt its very existence and think of it as a psychiatric problem, others regard it as a widespread disease that is dramatically underdiagnosed. In the United States, 3 to 5 percent of the population is allegedly affected, mostly women. The patients suffer from fatigue, low muscle strength, insomnia, headaches, and a lack of attentiveness. These symptoms might mean that the affected people need exercise. But it is also conceivable that this feebleness is a consequence of the disease. Fibromyalgia is diagnosed on the basis of 18 so-called tender points on the body. These points cannot be recognized anatomically but apparently hurt a little bit when you press on them.

The therapy options for fibromyalgia appear as arbitrary as the cause is mysterious. In Europe, some doctors put their patients in a warm mud bath, others try a medical cold chamber, but neither approach seems to work. Yet one treatment is emerging: in four studies looking into the effects of endurance training, physical exercise appears to allay the symptoms appreciably. As the fitness became better, the unusual fibromyalgia pain eased. Apparently, getting active helps the patients overcome their sickness because the newly gained muscle strength chases off fatigue, reduces pain, and helps patients handle their daily routine again—thus lifting up their spirits.[14]

HOPE FOR CHRONIC FATIGUE

Another complex of symptoms is known as Chronic Fatigue Syndrome (CFS), and it is also very mysterious. As with fibromyalgia, some physicians do not believe its very existence, whereas others are alarmed and call it a very serious condition. The affected people themselves report severe physical and mental exhaustion. If it lasts for six months or longer, and if it is accompanied by sleeping disorders, headache, and muscle weakness, the criteria for a CFS diagnosis are met. CFS was once thought to be caused by viruses, but no one has ever proven this.

This peculiar disease has attracted the interest of exercise researchers. CFS patients may simply be in poor physical shape. On the other hand, MRI imaging indicates that CFS patients have a defective muscle tissue—the oxygen consumption seems to be hampered.[15] The findings encouraged English doctors to analyze the impact of exercise on this illness. During the course of 12 weeks, CFS patients were asked to walk, bicycle, or swim regularly. Fatigue levels were indeed reduced as the patients got in better shape. Even a year after the study, these positive effects still lasted.[16]

INACTIVITY AND OSTEOPOROSIS

Of all women age 50 or older, about 20 percent are said to have fragile bones. This statement is based upon bone densitometry, a procedure that pharmaceutical companies, medical instrument-makers, and some pharmacists and gynecologists recommend.

The densitometry is usually carried out through X-rays. The denser the bone tissue, the more the X-rays are attenuated, which can be analyzed with a computer. The results are then compared to the standard bone density of a healthy 35-year-old human. An individual is said to have osteoporosis when her or his readings are 20 to 35 percent below an arbitrary threshold value (which equals 2.5 or more so-called standard deviations under the norm). This measuring system produces results that—if universally applied—would turn the vast majority of older people into osteoporosis patients—and at the same time into consumers for drugs that allegedly increase the density of the bones.

This whole concept would be a great idea, if it reached the actual goal: cutting down the number of broken bones. Alas, there is no reason to believe that that would be the case. Day after day, older people suffer from fractures—even when their bone density measurements produce perfectly normal values. Fifty to 70 percent of the osteoporosis-like fractures actually occur in women showing only a small deficiency in bone density.[17]

There is an abundance of studies indicating that women who participate in bone densitometries do not benefit at all. Researchers in Sweden, Germany, and the United States have come to this conclusion in independent trials. Over ten years ago experts at the British Columbia Office of Health Technology Assessment, in Vancouver, presented a thorough report on the question of whether diagnosing osteoporosis makes sense at all. Their conclusion: "Research evidence does not support either whole population or selective bone mineral density (BMD) testing of well women at or near menopause as a means to predict future fractures."[18] Consequently, health providers in countries like Germany have stopped paying for this useless procedure.

Drugs for osteoporosis have been shown to have no noteworthy clinical effect. The blockbuster is a substance called Alendronate, with annual sales of about $3 billion. The product's molecules migrate into the bone tissue and raise its density. In one study, women with an average age of 68 took the drug for four years, and the risk of hip fractures was allegedly reduced by 56 percent.[19]

Yet the American physician and author John Abramson took a closer look at the study; he was curious about what this number actually meant.[20] How many fractures of the hip were actually averted? The older participants who did not take the drug had a 99.5 percent chance of living one year without a hip fracture (among 1000 women, 995 would stay healthy). Among the women who actually took the drug, that chance was 99.8 percent (among 1000 women, 998 would stay healthy). In other words, the daily consumption of the drug changed the risk for a fracture from 0.5 to 0.2 percent. In the study, this modest result was boasted as a relative risk reduction of 56 percent.

Translated into real life, the drug's benefit looks like this: 81 women with low bone density must take the drug for 4.2 years (at a total cost of $300,000) in order to avoid *one* hip fracture.[21] Not only is this effect dearly paid for, there are also indications that it vanishes with time anyway. While a ten-year trial with the substance showed that the value of the bone density was increased, there was no proof that the risk of fractures had gone down—although that was the reason for this pharmacological intervention.[22]

But if the drug increases bone density, why is it not preventing fractures? Alendronate may increase bone density, but the bone density is, at best, only an indirect indicator of stability. The basic method for measuring the bone density, densitometry, targets the surface of the bone (the cortical bone). However, it is the inner structure (the trabecular bone) that mainly determines the stability of the big bones. Unfortunately, substances like Alendronate have a much greater effect on cortical bones than on trabecular bones. Thus, the pharmacological effect increases the reading for the bone density—yet the stability of the bones is not considerably increased.

In reality, there are other factors that influence the risk of fracture to a much greater extent. More important, for example, are the motor functions of older people and their ability to walk safely. Ninety-five to 98 percent of all fractures among older people occur because of a fall. In fact, it might be more suitable to talk about a "falling-down disease" rather than osteoporosis. Other key factors are the mass of the bone and its geometrical shape. In the United States, one out of three adults 65 years old or older falls each year, with hip fractures resulting in the greatest number of related deaths and serious health problems. Women account for 80 percent of the 300,000 hip fractures that occur annually.

In contrast to the bone density (which is weight per volume), the absolute bone mass indicates how much bone substance a human actually has. The bone mass peaks in young adulthood, and thereafter declines with age. In rare cases this loss is, for genetic reasons, extremely pronounced and hard to stop. Those affected may become hunchbacks relatively early in life.

Ordinarily, bone density is most determined by an environmental factor: exercise. Whenever we use our muscles, they, by exerting strain, increase the bone mass. Thus, in most cases osteoporosis is not a fateful disorder of bone metabolism but simply the direct result of decades of physical inactivity. And where gynecologists and employees of pharmaceutical companies blame menopausal changes as the cause of osteoporosis, they divert attention from the more important reason for the problem and conceal the most efficient remedy.

The muscular system has been found to determine 80 percent of bone stability. It was the German anatomist and surgeon Julius Wolff (1836–1902) who proposed this in his "law of the bone transformation," now known as Wolff's law. This law says that bones in a healthy person will adapt to the strains they are placed under. If loading on a particular bone increases, the bone will remodel itself over time to become stronger.

In the 1960s, the American orthopedist Harold M. Frost expanded this theory by emphasizing that muscles and bones comprise a single physiological unit: He proposed that the body must have specific sensors capable of recognizing mechanical forces and of relaying this information so that the bone grows according to this load. Whereas strain during muscle training triggers the growth of bone tissue, physical inactivity leads to loss of bone tissue.

Eckhard Schönau at the University Hospital in Cologne, Germany, along with colleagues, recently confirmed this hypothesis using CT imaging. The researchers put 349 healthy children and adolescents in CT scanners and determined precisely the composition of their bones and muscles. The data from this high-tech measurement fitted nicely into the old law of muscle transformation, and indeed suggested that the muscular system had determined the makeup of the bones. The sensors that Harold M. Frost had proposed as the reason for this were also discovered: bone cells are connected to each other by dendrites, and the resulting vast network can sense physical strain and adapt to it.[23]

The process of bone development begins early. An unborn baby, kicking away inside his mother's womb, gives his bones the mechanical strain needed to grow properly. Children need no advice to run and tumble and play; all that perpetual activity promotes the development of robust and healthy bones.

Neither milk nor calcium pills can substitute for exercise. A normal diet does contain enough calcium, but the body will flush it out swiftly if a person is not in motion. If you want the calcium to become part of your bones, you just have to heed Wolff's law and start using your muscles.

Actually the situation with osteoporosis drugs is quite similar. They can be beneficial for patients with severe loss of bone substance because they alleviate pain. Yet unless the consumption of the pills is accompanied with physical activity, they cannot compensate for the consequences of letting the body waste away.

Time and again, trials of menopausal women have confirmed that moderate aerobic and strength training make the spine stronger. And in order to reduce hip fractures, walking seems to be the best medicine. A study at Brigham and Women's Hospital in Boston, which included investigators from the Harvard School of Public Health, showed that women who walked at least four hours per week had approximately 40 percent fewer hip fractures, compared with women who were mostly sedentary. Higher-impact exercise provided greater protection. Exercise equivalent to about three hours of jogging per week reduced the risk of hip fracture by approximately 50 percent. "The news about walking continues to be positive, and our study contributes further evidence that regular physical activity is a woman's key to prevention of hip fractures," said Diane Feskanich of Brigham and Women's. "To reduce risk, women should know that any amount of activity is better than none."[24]

A team of researchers at the University of Freiburg, Germany, were curious whether they could make frail people more sure-footed again and tested this idea with a specific exercise for balance and agility.[25] Twenty volunteers from ages 60 to 80 practiced standing on one foot as they walked over wobbly planks and balanced on a rope on the floor. In their childhoods, these individuals would have laughed about how easy these tasks were—but now, after decades of nonuse of their bodies, they had to relearn these movements from scratch. At the end of the trial, the balance of participants was tested with clever tricks. They stood on a mat that would suddenly be pulled to one side and ran on a treadmill that was suddenly stopped. In comparison to those who had remained sedentary controls, the rate of tripping and losing balance was significantly reduced. This regained control over the motor skills is a good protection against falls.[26]

A survey in the United States compared the effectiveness of exercise with that of osteoporosis drugs. The study included 10,000 women over 65 and followed them for five years. The analysis of the data revealed that women who had trained for at least two hours per week had 36 percent fewer hip fractures than sedentary women, according to the journal *Annals of Internal Medicine*.[27] In the course of one year, there were six fewer fractures per 1,000 women among the active group of women than among the inactive ones. This effect is actually twice as big as the one reported in the aforementioned study on Alendronate.

The only effective way to keep bones in good shape is to stay active for life. Research shows it is never too late—getting started at age 80 is better than never. Mobilizing of a body also improves balance and makes one sure-footed, which is very important because falls, as we saw, are the main reason for bone fractures among elderly people. Moderate strength training, for example, is a good way to avoid falls. Tai chi creates awareness and body control, thus also reducing the likelihood of falls in older age.

The trial results discussed here have led to a turning point in orthopedics that would have seemed unthinkable just a short while ago. Physical motion was traditionally believed to be the worst thing one could inflict on an aching joint—until the opposite turned out to be true.

Unfortunately, the new knowledge about the healing power of exercise has not reached all people suffering from aching joints and bones. At the same time, in a sedentary and aging population, the number of muscular-skeletal diseases is increasing to the extent that physicians wonder if treating all the resulting ailments is financially possible. But when orthopedists gathered recently at a conference in Berlin, they agreed on the culprit of all of these maladies, saying that physical inactivity is the number-one public health problem of the third millennium.[28]

8

A Sporting Cure for Back Pain

James Weinstein reached forward to lift a heavy box. Suddenly, he felt an extraordinary pain shooting through his back. Weinstein, a silver-haired professor, was unable to sit down, but somehow he managed to lie on the floor and rest. When Weinstein tried to get up after a while, it took a tremendous struggle.

Thousands of individuals all over the United States are in a similarly miserable situation at any given moment. From one second to the next, the world is a different place. It's as if a glowing dagger were prodding the lumbar vertebrae. Happy people turn into creatures of misery.

But Weinstein immediately knew what to do. He is one of the most renowned back specialists in the United States and teaches at Dartmouth Medical School in Hanover, New Hampshire. Weinstein took an anti-inflammatory drug, put ice on the aching spot—and went jogging.[1]

This approach borders on heresy. People suffering from acute pain are usually asked to rest at least until the pain has markedly abated or completely disappeared. Yet the ailing professor merely heeded the advice he gives patients in his own back-pain program at Dartmouth: Hurt does not mean harm. "In other words, one can have pain and still function."[2]

Weinstein is not the only physician to discover that exercise is the key to overcoming lower back pain and triggering the body's power to heal itself. Increasingly, doctors encourage back-pain patients to stay active and to soldier on with their daily routines.

What a complete turnabout this is! Just a few years ago, people with lower-back pain were prescribed strict bed rest lasting one to two weeks. Afterward, they were ordered to take it easy and to avoid everything that would cause discomfort. However, a few physicians started to rebel against the common wisdom and demanded exactly the opposite. Patients suffering from lower-back pain, they thought, should stay physically active.

The British doctor Gordon Waddell was one of the first to question these contradicting approaches and tried to determine which one was right. He and two of his colleagues carried out a unique survey, analyzing all the scientific papers they could find that studied the effects of either bed rest, or an active recovery, on lower-back pain. It turned out that bed rest led to terrible outcomes. Consequently, Waddell and his colleagues wrote a paper demanding a radical reversal of the traditional bed-rest treatment: "A simple but fundamental change from the traditional prescription of bed rest to positive advice about staying active could improve clinical outcomes and reduce the personal and social impact of back pain."[3] In the wake of this revelation, medical guidelines and official recommendations gradually dropped the principle of complete rest.

Yet in many consultations, these revised recommendations are forgotten. This is particularly worrisome given that the mind-set and advice of a physician profoundly influences the development of an individual sickness. The general practitioner Annette Becker, of the University Hospital in Marburg, Germany, writes, "Thoughtless remarks or putative explanations like ascribing problems to 'wear and tear,' recommending rest, or repeated passive measures like massages and giving sick notes to exempt patients from certain obligations trigger, especially among fearful and dramatizing patients, only more worries about their well-being, like: 'I must be careful with my back, I've worked too much in my life, I must think about myself now.'" This type of thinking can lead to a vicious circle. Individuals with chronic back pain stop using their bodies and slide into complete inactivity. Their backs continue to waste away, which triggers new waves of pain.[4]

SORE BACK TODAY, DISABLED TOMORROW?

At any given time, about 35 to 40 percent of the adult population in the industrialized countries suffer from back pain. Fortunately, in most cases these aches disappear by themselves. But about 10 percent of the time the pain stays, and becomes chronic. And about 5 percent of all back patients turn into problem cases: following their back spasm, "lumbago," or a slipped disk, they never become fully functional people again. They are unable to work, are deemed disabled, and their back pain governs their lives.[5]

The sad fact that millions of patients have suffered through all this is caused in part by an incorrect view that still persists in the medical world. Traditionally many doctors regard back pain as a mechanical problem: If there is pain, there must be a physical problem. But this way of thinking can have adverse consequences: The patients are examined over and over with increasingly aggressive methods, until the doctor makes a diagnosis and starts a treatment that, in reality, is not related to the pain.[6]

The mechanical trigger of back pain is a phantom that has been chased by medical professionals for more than 100 years. During this hunt, many theories have become dominant, only to be quickly abandoned. Once, flatfeet were thought to cause back pain. In turn, gout, festered maxillary sinuses, syphilis, colds, and varicose veins have all been said to be the culprit. And because the prevalence of back pain seemed to rise during the nineteenth century, when the first railway networks were built, the so-called railway spine syndrome became the disease of the day. According to this idea, back pain was triggered not only by severe injuries but also by the minor bumps and shaking caused by the speed of moving trains.

In 1934, the American physicians William Mixter and Joseph Barr developed the theory further and announced that slipped and damaged disks caused back pain. By 1945, this dogma held that disks caused 99 percent of all back-pain cases. Subsequently, back surgery took off, and continues booming to this day. Medical historians coined the term "dynasty of the disk," and the surgical removal of a disk (discectomy) is today one of the standard procedures in orthopedics.

At first glance, this all makes perfect sense. The processes going on between the disks of our spine seem designed for disaster. Surprisingly early in life, disks are prone to fissures, wearing down, and loosening. By the time we are 20, the tissue of the disk has become worn down and tends to protrude or prolapse. When the orthopedist Jürgen Krämer headed the International Society for the Study of the Lumbar Spine, his presidential address was on the natural course of disk diseases: "The degeneration curve starts at the age of one when humans begin to squeeze their discs in the upright position. Disc degeneration is progressive and almost universal in the human spine. The curve ends up with 100 percent disk degeneration in the aging spine."[7]

This decline is caused by the biological composition of the disks. Made of a gelatinous type of tissue, they are not supplied by blood vessels and absorb nutrition as a sponge does. While we are sitting and standing, these disks become squeezed, so that fluids containing waste material can leave the disk tissue. Yet while we are lying down, disks take in fluids and become saturated with all the nutrients they need. "The disc," says Krämer, "is an osmotic system that lives on motion. Because of the human sedentary nonmoving lifestyle, disc generation is progressive."

By now, all these degenerative processes in the spine can be detected by CT and MRI scans in greater detail than ever before. But that is not necessarily good for the patient. When doctors examine individuals who have no pain at all and consider their backs to be healthy, they usually come up with alarming results. In one trial, 67 volunteers with no history of back problems were scanned by MRI.[8] Among the subjects under the age of 60, it was found that one in five actually had at least one disk prolapse. In one out of two cases, there was a protrusion of at least one disk. The results for the subjects at age 60 or older looked even worse: More than 30 percent had a disk prolapse, and nearly 80 percent had a protruded disk. And yet all those people were not in pain. The renowned specialist Richard Deyo at Harborview Medical Center in Seattle states: "Detecting a herniated disk on an imaging test therefore proves only one thing conclusively: the patient has a herniated disk."[9]

As long as an individual with a disk prolapse is free of pain, he or she will not usually have surgery. However, if doctors encounter a person with pain and a herniated disk at the same time, both physician and patient are convinced they have found the reason for the pain. The orthopedist Steffen Heger says: "Two events happen at the same time in a patient, consequently a casual relation is postulated."[10]

Yet in many cases such a correlation is not a given. When a person has a slipped disk, it is not necessarily the cause of the pain. Nevertheless, such a patient is very likely to have surgery, says Heger: "One must assume that in many cases something was operated on that wasn't the cause of the back pain."

Small wonder so many patients feel little or no real alleviation after surgery. According to various studies, 10 to 60 percent of all operations fail in this way. These unnecessary procedures are so numerous that they have given rise to a new medical condition: the "failed back surgery syndrome."

When patients suffering from lower back pain are examined, in 85 percent of the cases the resulting diagnosis does not actually reveal what causes the pain. The association between symptoms and the results of the imaging is weak, and many doctors like to say strain or sprains were the trouble-makers. Yet "strain and sprain have never been anatomically or histologically characterized, and patients given these diagnoses might accurately be said to have idiopathic low back pain."[11]

The still-widespread belief that physical damage to a disk is behind all back pain is the main reason so many doctors continue to regard bed rest as a therapeutic measure. The well-intentioned result is often that a person suffering from back pain takes time off work and goes to bed. Yet more up-to-date experts agree that it is just this immobilization that can turn aches into chronic pain. "Bed rest doesn't only weaken the muscular system but it also leads on to inactivity osteoporosis," says Heger. Psychologists also believe bed rest is dramatically underestimated as a trigger of sickness and that "the prescription of too long bed rest is one of the principal reasons for physical deconditioning."[12]

Here again we see the danger of going to bed: Only 50 percent of all back patients who have been off work longer than six months ever make it back to their jobs.

THE CULPRIT: DETERIORATING MUSCLES

Cartilage, ligaments, and bones are not the only components that help to keep the back in shape and give us good posture; muscles also play a key role in stabilizing the body. Although they enable our back to move, they also restrain it, like a corset, with the flexibility needed in our back to absorb shocks. This way, jerky movements and falls usually do not result in slipped or ruptured disks.

There are two parts to our musculature with different tasks. The *global* system consists of long muscles usually located at the surface of the body. They make possible the movements of the body. By contrast, the muscles of the *local* system are short, run transversely to the body, and are close to the joints. This way, they support the joints and protect them against sudden movements and mechanical overload. This muscle corset is the precondition for a strong and trouble-free back. The stability of the lumbar spine, for example, is 80 percent due to muscles.[13] Losing this stability is a major reason for acute and chronic back pain.

Despite the key role of muscles, the standard diagnostic tests for lower-back pain almost always involve the disks and the vertebrae. The shape and the composition of the muscle system, on the other hand, are often not examined at all. Fortunately, some physicians have developed a model that takes all the components into account. This includes the passive system, composed of bones, ligaments, and joints; and the active system, consisting of muscles. This comprehensive model is important because the active and the passive systems depend on each other, and each is able to compensate for deficiencies in the other system. Also, muscles can be reactivated, even after decades of nonuse, and are a proven remedy for overcoming back pain.

An example for a stabilizing muscle is the *Musculus transversus abdominis*, lying in the deepest layer of the stomach muscles. Another one is the *Musculus multifidus*, which connects the transverse processes (*Processus transversi*) of the vertebrae with the spinous processes (*Processus spinosus*). It straightens up the back and gives us good posture. This and other muscles, as well as bones and ligaments, act together and usually keep the spine from being twisted and destabilized.

Yet it's important that the muscles of the global system also remain in good shape. There are some muscles that act as "global mobilizers" and are needed to carry heavy weights, like the rectus abdominis muscle (*Musculus rectus abdominis*) and the extensors along the spine. The better they are at this job, the more they help the system of local muscles. Consequently, the local muscles can be used more exclusively to protect and stabilize the spine. This means that people suffering from back pain should make sure their system of global muscles systems is in adequate shape, especially if they have to lift heavy weights at work or at home.[14]

The more the muscles waste away, the faster bones, ligaments, and disks lose their protection. Trials measuring the muscle strength of people suffering from back pain have confirmed that both aspects are closely related. The longer the pain persisted, the weaker the back extensors became. One study compared patients who had gone through back surgery with healthy people: The average maximum strength of the back patients was 40 percent lower. Furthermore, individuals with ailing backs were found to have below-average strength leg muscles as well as an asymmetric distribution of muscles along the torso, a recipe for more back spasms. In the end, a spine can end up downright twisted.

The back muscles of patients with chronic back pain are not only feebler than those of normal people; they also tire more quickly. This becomes clear when patients are asked to work out: after a fairly small number of repetitions, they are simply unable to keep up. In several studies this failure was shown to be caused by degenerative processes on the cellular level; these individuals have more type-II muscles than usual, which wear out rapidly.

MENDING THE MIND, MENDING THE BACK

Often, the sore back and the decline of muscle strength are accompanied by a decline in mental health. Some people even become accustomed to the idea of living the rest of their lives as a disabled back patient.

The physician Jan Hildebrandt and the psychologist Michael Pfingsten have examined many severe back cases at their center in the University Hospital in Göttingen, Germany, and have noticed that the amount and intensity of pain is not determined by pathological changes in the back and its muscles. Rather, the way a patient *thinks* about his sickness predicts how much pain he will feel. Many back-pain patients are deeply convinced they are handicapped—even when doctors and therapists offer a good prognosis.[15]

Many patients even stop working and try to live on disability benefits because it appears to all to be the most convenient solution. The employer gets rid of the employee who is always sick and complaining; the doctor has one less whining patient.

Yet this is not the way things have to end. The new science of healing through exercise shows that even the most desperate patients have reason to be optimistic. To start with, disk material that slipped into the epidural space is recognized as a foreign body and is often attacked and destroyed by the body's own enzymes. Physical exercise also seems to promote the healing of damaged tissue.[16] Degenerative changes affecting the back and stomach muscles can be systematically reversed. Regardless of how neglected and atrophied muscle cells are, training can awaken these sleeping beauties and give them new strength and endurance.

In order to reap these benefits, patients just have to have confidence in the scientific facts: Exercise and strain do no harm but are needed if the back is to heal. Treating chronic back pain with only pain relievers is not enough, although sometimes drugs might be necessary to help patients start a therapeutic exercise program.[17]

Patients who stay with it find that seemingly miraculous changes often start to occur after a few days of training. As they begin using their muscles again, their fear of "putting their back out" due to an unfortunate movement diminishes. As a result, their moods brighten and a chance opens up to escape the vicious cycle of chronic pain and physical inactivity.

Hildebrandt and Pfingsten have shown hundreds of patients that it is indeed possible to overcome the pain. They have developed a four-week program consisting of aerobic endurance training, games, swimming, strength training, relaxation exercises, and psychotherapy. They have tested their program among patients who were already medically declared unable to work and given negative psychiatric diagnoses.

Their results? Even the most problematic patients had improvements. Mentally, patients appeared much happier. They had less pain and less depression and looked ahead with more confidence. Physically, measurements showed that their torso muscles became stronger.

Interestingly, most patients did not think the psychotherapy part of the program was crucial to their success. Rather, they regarded their dramatically increased muscle strength and greatly improved endurance as turning points in their medical history. A new awareness of their own bodies emerged, and their fear of hurting their backs was lowered. After going through this program, 63 percent of the patients were able to resume their jobs and daily lives.[18]

Surgeons would be happy if they achieved such a success rate. There is no doubt that in many instances an injured back needs an operation, for instance, when patients lose control over sphincter and bladder. This usually signals that a massive prolapse has compressed the nerves in the pelvic region. When these muscles fail to work, when a foot cannot be moved, or when other body parts become inoperative, most doctors agree it is high time for surgery. In other cases, when back pain and fever occur at the same time, there might be an inflammation rampaging near the spine. Finally, there even might be a tumor growing and compressing nerves in the back.

Although these and other conditions require surgical treatment, most surgical procedures are advised to alleviate pain and prevent further progression of the problem. But what is the outcome of the surgical removal, in part or whole, of an intervertebral disk? The experts James Weinstein, Richard Deyo, and colleagues compared the outcomes of surgical and nonsurgical treatment in a randomized study that included more than 500 women and men in 13 spine clinics in 11 U.S. states.[19] One-half of the patients underwent discectomy; the other half received nonsurgical treatments like physical therapy, education with some home exercise instructions, and anti-inflammatory drugs.

After two years, the outcome revealed that patients with herniated disks improved whether they had surgery or not. Though surgery appeared to alleviate pain faster, on average all patients had gotten better, and there was no substantial difference between the two groups.

This is significant because in many cases physicians pressure patients by telling them that, without surgery, their conditions will worsen. Now, the first study about this question reveals this is not the case at all. Eugene Carragee of Stanford University Medical Center in California states: "The fear of many patients and surgeons that not removing a large disk herniation will likely have catastrophic neurological consequences is simply not borne out."[20]

A similarly cautious approach appears appropriate when doctors press for another sort of back surgery, spinal-fusion surgery. During this procedure, which is rapidly increasing in the United States, physicians use metal screws and rods to fuse two or more vertebrae. Though this complex and risky intervention has been performed for 90 years, it was only a few years ago that researchers set out to analyze its success.

The trial, led by Jeremy Fairbank at the Nuffield Orthopaedic Centre in Oxford, involved 349 chronic back pain patients. Of these, 176 were assigned to spinal-fusion surgery and 173 to a three-week intensive program of rehabilitation, involving daily exercises and cognitive behavioral therapy. The rehabilitation aimed not only to address physical ailments but also to help patients overcome fear of pain or exercise, to learn to cope with the psychological effects of pain, and to learn to relax.

There appeared to be a slight advantage to surgical treatment, but the difference was barely significant in clinical terms. Thus, Fairbank states: "There was no clear evidence from our trial that primary spinal fusion surgery was more beneficial than intensive rehabilitation. Our results suggest that patients eligible for surgery should be offered a rehabilitation program first. We believe it is safer and cheaper than using surgery as the first line of treatment."[21]

If a patient, as is so often the case, still feels pain and discomfort after surgery for a herniated disk, these complaints do not necessarily result in self-doubt and restraint among surgeons. Frequently they will recommend a second operation, especially if they are not responsible for the first. In these cases doctors like to say their colleagues have just bungled the operations, whereas the next surgery, usually a spinal fusion, will fix the whole mess.[22]

But is a second surgery better than exercise? Recently, Norwegian researchers carried out a trial to answer this question.[23] The study surveyed 60 patients who were in miserable condition, all with lower-back pain lasting longer than a year, despite undergoing—or because they had undergone—disk surgery.

The participants were randomly divided into two groups. In the first one, experienced back surgeons performed fusions. In the second one, the participants were taught that ordinary physical activity would not harm their disks. They also received tips on how to use their backs and how to bend and had exercise sessions for three weeks, with three sessions per day. One year later, Jens Ivar Brox of the Medical Faculty University in Oslo and his colleagues measured the outcome by questioning the participants about their pain and related disability.

Fifty percent of the fusion group reported improvements, compared to 48 percent in the exercise group—hardly a substantial difference. The researchers concluded that patients should beware of the scalpel: "Our interpretation of the present evidence is that lumbar fusion should not be recommended in patients with chronic low back pain after surgery for disc herniation."[24]

AEROBICS FOR A FIT BACK

Programs for making disabled back patients fit and mobile again need not be sophisticated and expensive. This is the conclusion of a trial that Swiss doctors carried out with 148 patients who suffered for more than three months from low-back pain serious enough to require medical attention or absence from work.[25] The participants were randomly assigned to three groups: the first had physiotherapy, the second trained their muscles on exercise machines, and the third participated in ordinary aerobics classes. Each program lasted for three months, with two sessions per week. Using questionnaires, at four different intervals, the researchers assessed how their patients were doing: before and after the program, and 6 and 12 months later.

There were many improvements. In all groups, participants reported the pain level remained substantially reduced, even after 12 months. This long-lasting effect is apparently because 80 percent of the patients continued with their respective exercises after the official end of the three-month program. Fear of injury was reduced in all three groups and stayed on a lower level up to the 12-month follow-up.

The one exception to this continuing success was in the level of disability. Over the course of the three-month program, the level went down for all groups. However, this effect was soon lost among the patients who had done physiotherapy. Evidently, once they could no longer go to the therapist, these patients were unable to overcome their fear of injury. The researchers concluded: "One-to-one physiotherapy perhaps promotes a sense of dependence of the patient on the therapist to guide and govern the most appropriate activity level for them in accordance with their declared level of pain."[26] By contrast, participants in the muscle-training group and the aerobics group fared much better and continued to feel less impaired following the program.

This study, reported in the journal *Rheumatology*, has important repercussions: aerobics classes in an ordinary gym are as effective as weight training for treating back ailments, and in the long term both approaches appear superior to physiotherapy. The latter two procedures are relatively expensive, whereas aerobics classes in Europe are cheaper and thus advocated by the researchers: "The introduction of low-impact aerobic exercise programs for patients with [chronic low-back pain] should allow considerable savings in the direct costs associated with its treatment."[27]

The aerobics classes were likely successful because they cured the patients' fears of using their bodies. This would confirm the insight of James Weinstein, after he wrenched his own back. When he came back from his run, Weinstein felt "pretty good."[28]

9

Exercise and Brain Power

A HEALTHY BABY IS BORN WITH 160 TO 180 BILLION NERVE CELLS in his or her brain, and in the first four years of life, this lavish endowment will transform into a finished brain, with an average of only slightly more than 100 billion nerve cells. In these early years, while the brain downsizes and develops at the same time, it is extremely important that a child has sufficient physical exercise. Good coordination of the body helps to preserve nerve cells in the brain and promotes their wiring to each other.[1] Evidence indicates children need a certain minimum amount of exercise to develop a brain malleable or plastic enough to adapt to ever-changing environments.

Not long ago, this connection between physical and mental skills was disputed. Psychologists and psychiatrists thought that motor activity and cognitive performance resided in two distinct realms. This concept lives on in the terms anatomists use to describe the brain. On one side is the cerebellum, traditionally depicted as the brain's center for motor activity, which is in charge of the learning of movements. On the other side is the prefrontal cortex, long seen as the center for cognitive tasks like planning and behavior in social groups.

The domains for motor activity and cognition were also thought to be separate for chronological reasons. The development of motor skills, it was thought, started early in life and was quickly completed. The development of the cognitive abilities, however, would follow later and would not be affected by physical exercise at all.

For a long time, it was thought that the brain was supplied with blood in a constant mode that could not be changed by external factors like exercise and training. It was not before the availability of novel brain imaging techniques that this assumption could be experimentally tested. Wildor Hollmann and colleagues of the German Sport University, Cologne, encouraged young and healthy students to train on stationary bikes. Using positron emission tomography (PET), the researchers monitored brain activity while the students were exercising. When the energy expended reached 25 watts, blood circulation in the brain increased on average by 20 percent, and at 100 watts the increase was 30 percent.

BUILDING THE BRAIN THROUGH MOTION

These data proved the idea of the physiologically separate brain wrong and revealed the opposite to be true: If a person exercises moderately, blood circulation within the gray matter increases substantially. Interestingly, studies of rats running on treadmills showed that this boost does not affect all parts of the brain equally. Although the blood supply is even reduced in some areas, it is greatly increased in others—which indicates that the bloodstream specifically transports nutrients and oxygen to certain brain areas. Insulin-like growth factor is among the substances taken up by nerve cells in these areas, making the cells excitable. Also, after just 30 minutes of running, certain proteins are produced in greater numbers within the nerve cells in some brain areas. And after running over a period of three months on treadmills, rats showed a distinct pattern: many genes and proteins critical for the functioning of the synapses between neurons and for the plasticity were activated.[2]

The proteins' nerve growth factor (NGF) and the brain-derived neurotrophic factor (BDNF) are also produced in great quantities in the brain when the body is exercising, and both act like brain fertilizers: if their levels are high, the nerve cells luxuriate. Furthermore, the blood level of the amino acid tryptophan rises in response to physical training. Tryptophan then leads to an increased production of the neurotransmitter serotonin. Finally, endorphins are also elevated by physical activity, and both substances act as mood enhancers. Doctors can use these beneficial brain chemicals by prescribing regular physical activity for depressed patients.

Physical activity not only enriches chemistry in the gray matter; it also alters the structure of the brain. First, exercise promotes the production of new nerve cells in the hippocampus. (We'll see later how much this fountain of youth influences our mental well-being and power.) Second, exercise creates new synapses, thereby establishing and maintaining the vast network of connected nerve cells in the brain. These many effects help optimize the intellectual development of children.

Surveys in preschools and elementary schools have confirmed this direct link. One trial in Cologne included 600 children from 12 elementary schools. The students were asked to run for six minutes, and the researchers documented the distance they covered. Another test concerned physical coordination. The children were encouraged to walk backward, to jump on one leg, and to move around a curve using crossover steps. A further test involved sorting and labeling certain symbols according to their importance. This measures the ability to pay attention, a fundamental cognitive skill.

The results: performance in the six-minute run did not actually correlate with results in the cognitive test. However, physical coordination was clearly linked to cleverness. The students with above-average motor activity were also superior in their ability to concentrate. Thus physical coordination and mental ability may reside in the same realm of the brain.

But how could that be? The researchers who carried out the study think it might be because the two skills are represented in overlapping brain areas. Thus activating certain parts of the brain by "motor activities 'trains' them possibly in such a way that they also function better in other situations, for example during work requiring mental concentration."[3]

Researchers from the International University in Bremen tested 85 boys and girls ages four to six and asked them to perform seven different tasks involving strength, physical flexibility, speed, and coordination. A further test measured their cognitive skills: the children had to spot certain differences in pictures, which measured their attention spans, memory, nonverbal intelligence, and other cognitive capabilities.

These results also show that cognitive and motor skills are connected. Well-coordinated children achieved above-average results in the picture test. These findings underline that the two kinds of development go hand in hand: The more time spent skipping rope, playing hopscotch, riding bicycles, climbing, walking to school, practicing gymnastics, and playing outdoors, the better. Claudia Voelcker-Rehage, lead author of the study, concludes that, especially among children aged four to five, development of coordination and cognition is linked, meaning that in preschools an "integrated stimulation for both cognition and motor activity is very important."[4]

Findings from brain scans analyzing the functional anatomy confirm that the two domains are indeed very closely connected. When the brain is working on a cognitive problem, areas of the prefrontal cortex are activated, and regions of the cerebellum *also* light up. A similar double pattern appears when the brain is trying to solve tasks related to language—for example, trying to say as many words as possible within one minute that start with the same letter. Conversely, as soon as the individual being tested has solved the problem and does not need to concentrate any longer, the activity patterns in both the prefrontal cortex and the cerebellum fade away.

People with damaged, malfunctioning cerebellums not only have impaired motor activities but often struggle when asked to solve cognitive tasks that involve planning, memorizing, and finding words. There are even speech disorders that are solely caused by pathologically low activity in the cerebellum.[5]

The process of learning to speak and write is another example revealing that mental and motor activities are linked. Even when babies or small children are unable to speak, they can already grasp the words they hear. But only when children have the motor skills to write by hand can they internalize the concept of scripted language. The motor activities connected with handwriting cannot be replaced by hitting keys on a computer keyboard. Rather, experts recommend children and their parents train the motor skills with activities like drawing, crafts, and also ball games.[6]

When such training does not occur, the motor skills may not fully develop, which in turn can result in cognitive impairments and disorders. Many children with dyslexia and related problems often also struggle to coordinate their movements. Adele Diamond, a neuroscientist at the University of British Columbia in Vancouver, states: "Children who are dyslexic, like children who are clumsy, have difficulties with continuous tapping tasks compared to same-aged peers."[7]

Among young people suffering from autism, impaired motor activities are also frequently seen. Interestingly, researchers believe autism is linked to a narrowed cerebellum as well as to a delayed maturation of the prefrontal cortex. The two areas seem to be so closely related that impairment in one area can cause a malfunctioning in the other.

GAMES, NOT PILLS, FOR ADHD

When they see restless and agitated children, many doctors are quick to diagnose a disease called attention deficit hyperactivity disorder (ADHD). Many claim that this disorder is genetically determined and should for this reason be treated with pharmacological substances like methylphenidate (Ritalin), which alter the metabolism of a child's brain.

ADHD's estimated worldwide prevalence in people under age 19 is about 5 percent, but there is enormous variability in estimates, and the United States has an especially high rate of ADHD, with 10 percent of males and 4 percent of females diagnosed with it. Thus, according to the statistics, in every classroom there are one or two fidgeting kids who need professional help. In recent years, many teachers and parents have arrived at the conclusion that ADHD is an innate disorder affecting the metabolism of the brain. But to this day there is no scientific method of telling the brain of a normal child from the brain of a child who is said to have ADHD.

Only with the aid of arbitrary criteria can a preschool child or young student be given the ADHD label. But the symptoms ("easily distracted," "doesn't sit still") are so random that they can be seen in a variety of forms among most children. It appears impossible to draw an objective line between a healthy temperament and disturbed behavior.

Methylphenidate was first synthesized in 1944 by a chemist, Leandro Panizzon, with the company Ciba.[8] He swallowed the substance in an experiment on himself but did not experience much from it. His wife, Marguerite—known as Rita—tried it, too, and felt a quite inspiring effect. From this time on Rita would consume the substance occasionally when she was getting ready for a tennis match, and it was named after her: Ritalin.

At first, Ritalin was given to adults only to treat depression, mental fatigue, and disorientation among elderly people. The disease that would make Ritalin famous, and notorious, had not yet been invented. It was not until the 1960s that research became public showing that methylphenidate, and a similar substance called dexedrine, had a quieting effect on children with learning difficulties. By now, methylphenidate is marketed in specific doses, some lasting 8 to 12 hours. The children who are told to take this drug at breakfast spend the full day under medication.

As the consumption of methylphenidate has exploded in industrialized countries, teens and young adults in the United States take the drug for additional reasons: as an appetite suppressant or to stave off the urge to sleep. They crush the tablets and snort the powder to get high. Youngsters have little difficulty obtaining methylphenidate from classmates or friends with prescriptions. The U.S. Drug Enforcement Administration has posted a drastic warning: "Methylphenidate, a Schedule II substance, has a high potential for abuse and produces many of the same effects as cocaine or the amphetamines. The abuse of this substance has been documented among narcotic addicts who dissolve the tablets in water and inject the mixture. Complications arising from this practice are common due to the insoluble fillers used in the tablets. When injected, these materials block small blood vessels, causing serious damage to the lungs and retina of the eye. Binge use, psychotic episodes, cardiovascular complications, and severe psychological addiction have all been associated with methylphenidate abuse."[9]

To this day, it is not known what methylphenidate actually does in the still-developing brain of a preschool or kindergarten child. Nora Volkow, now director of the National Institute on Drug Abuse in Rockville, Maryland, found that the substance, by blocking certain transporting proteins, increases the level of the neurotransmitter dopamine in the synapses, thus acting much like cocaine.[10] However, methylphenidate does not appear to be as addictive, given that it is ingested in pill form. It takes hold much more slowly than cocaine and does not create such a high.

Even when properly prescribed by a doctor, the consumption of the drug comes with a whole range of side effects: agitation, fear, sleeping problems, and paranoia. If the drug is dropped after a long-term treatment, there may be withdrawal symptoms. The drug can spoil a child's appetite.

Yet many parents are relieved when their child is diagnosed with ADHD because it unburdens them: If my child's problems are caused by an innate defect of brain chemistry, the thinking goes, the way we are raising our children is not involved. The label ADHD, however, has serious repercussions for children, who learn to think: I can only be tolerated by my parents and teachers when I take my drugs.

"The medication with regulating substances might be advisable for correcting some deficits or for starting an integral therapy," says Christina Hahn at the Institute of Sport and Sport Science of the University of Heidelberg, Germany. "As a child-oriented, long-ranging treatment, however, medication is by no means the only solution of the problem."[11]

Among children diagnosed with the syndrome, a familiar pattern appears. More than half of these children not only have problems concentrating but are conspicuously awkward; they are bad at balancing and have difficulties timing their movements. This could mean that exercises in improving coordination might be useful to improve concentration and attention.

Though problems with motor activity are not the main symptoms of ADHD, autism, and dyslexia, it is eye-catching that these problems appear so often along with impaired co-ordination. Adele Diamond concludes: "Motor development and cognitive development may be much more interrelated than has been previously appreciated. Indeed, they may be fundamentally intertwined."[12]

But physical training is nearly never prescribed; the rule instead is to give children medication. On any given day, hundreds of thousands of children are served tablets for breakfast to calm them down and make them attentive. In about 20 minutes the substance takes hold, and the children show a different behavior.

By contrast, prescribing sports programs for children with ADHD appears to be a much gentler and longer-lasting approach. Only a few researchers have developed specific exercise programs for inattentive children, and Gerd Hölter at the University of Dortmund, Germany, is one of them. In one trial, therapists, children, and their parents met once a week for three months in a swimming pool. While educators coached the parents, the children played in the water and tried things like diving for rings. After encouraging results, Hölter plans to expand his program by adding games in a gym. He says: "More exercise and behavioral therapy and less Ritalin—this is our concept."[13]

In the meantime, Hahn has already gathered scientific data documenting the beneficial influence of exercise on children diagnosed with ADHD. More than 90 children, mostly boys with an average age of eight and a half, participated in the study. At first, researchers tested motor skills and the ability to concentrate on problems. Some children were actually taking methylphenidate, and their parents were asked not to change the medication during the study so that the results would not be distorted.

The children were randomly assigned to three groups. Members of the first one played ball games most of the time, soccer and field hockey, learning techniques and tactics. That way, the researchers aimed to simulate how children played in the 1950s and 1960s when it was normal for them to spend summer days outside, playing in yards and fields. The participants of the second group rode mountain bikes, learned in-line skating, and took climbing lessons. Both sports programs lasted 90 minutes and took place twice a week. The third group was used as a control, with 37 ADHD-diagnosed children who did not play any sports at all.

Six months later, Hahn and her colleagues retested the motor skills and concentration abilities of the children. The sedentary children had largely the same results as at the beginning of the study, and there was even further deterioration to be seen, possibly an adverse effect of the methylphenidate some of the children continued to take. The drugs slow down the natural desire to move and thus impair the motor skills all the more.

By contrast, the children in both sports groups did much better. Although their motor skills were markedly subpar at the beginning of the study, they improved dramatically and even reached the lower range of what is considered normal. Their ability to concentrate also improved greatly. These budding athletes solved more cognitive problems than the controls in a given time.[14]

These results confirm what the findings of the neuroscientists suggest: If we train our motor abilities by exercising, at the same time we strengthen regions of the brain that are important for paying attention and other cognitive capabilities. Playing sports makes us smarter, and all children can benefit from this effect—whether they are diagnosed with an attention disorder or not.

10

Lifting the Spirit

A BLEAK MIND AND A LIFE FULL OF ACTIVITY? THESE TWO THINGS DO not seem to match. Sedentary people tend to have a heavy heart, and sad people are often physically inactive. The correlation is so stable and widespread that it has been demonstrated in many epidemiological trials. Study after study has shown that the more we utilize our muscles, the more positive feelings develop in our heads. This also applies to latecomers to exercise: if a person gets going in advanced age, the risk of developing depression drops to the low levels enjoyed by people who have been active from early on in life. The reverse strategy cannot be recommended. Formerly active people who refrain from using their muscles in middle age have a higher likelihood of developing psychiatric problems.

Although this relationship has been known since the 1980s, psychiatrists and psychologists have just started to use the healing power of exercise in the treatment of mental disorders. In contrast to cardiologists, they largely disregarded the influence of regular exercise on mental well-being.[1] Some psychiatrists believe it is high time to alter this attitude: "The clinical psychiatry of the recent past and present with its focus on psychotherapy and pharmacotherapy regards sports and games rather as simply a fine pastime and doesn't so far attribute any specific therapeutic effectiveness to it."[2]

The reservations shown by many psychologists and psychiatrists in this regard are even more astonishing given that there is now a wealth of data indicating specifically that people suffering from depression and anxiety disorders benefit from physical exercise. Multiple studies also show that more than just psychiatric impairments can be successfully treated with training. Neurodegenerative disorders like Alzheimer's disease, characterized by dramatic losses of brain mass and nerve cells, are being studied in relation to physical activity. These diseases, once they develop, are curable with neither tablets nor training. Yet exercise appears to be one of the best means to prevent them from developing in the first place.

FROM THE COUCH TO THE TREADMILL

Only a few patients who suffer from depression become healthy again by taking drugs. About 65 to 75 percent of those patients who do so are not cured and have to face recurring depressive episodes: they are sad, easily agitated, and have problems sleeping and concentrating. This is due not only to the fact that drugs have little effect, but it is also because up to 60 percent of patients are believed to stop following their prescriptions after three weeks. Others refuse to take antidepressants in the first place for fear of being stigmatized.

In the face of all these problems, some doctors started to wonder whether there might be a better alternative. Ideally this would be a remedy that is effective, has no adverse side effects, and is socially accepted. Older studies among healthy subjects had indicated that physical exercise is an ideal candidate to fit this description. Endurance training had been found to lighten moods, reduce fears, and increase the capacity to cope with stress. In one study, groups of active and sedentary people were followed for eight years, with the conclusion being that inactive people developed a depression rate twice that of their active counterparts.

Other trials included patients suffering from mild to severe depression. In one study, 40 patients were encouraged either to participate in a running program for eight weeks or to try strength training for eight weeks. Tests before and after the program revealed improved symptoms in both groups.[3]

Does that mean exercise beats pharmaceuticals in terms of effectiveness? The research group of James Blumenthal at Duke Medical Center in Durham, North Carolina, set out to answer this question.[4] They randomly assigned 156 elderly patients, who suffered from major depression, into three groups: those exercising, those taking antidepressants (in this case sertraline hydrochloride, which is an antidepressant of the selective serotonin reuptake inhibitor class), and those trying both. The exercise session lasted for 30 minutes, three days per week.

After 16 weeks, the participants were reexamined. In all three groups, the patients' health had significantly improved, and about 60 percent of each group were no longer depressed.

Therefore the program relying solely on physical activity was as effective as state-of-the-art antidepressants.

Over time, the effect of exercise became more pronounced. The participants were examined after six months, and those on exercise regimens had significantly fewer relapses than the drug-takers. The long-lasting effect of activity can be explained by the fact that many of the participants liked exercising so much that they continued to be active even after the official end of the study. That way, they overcame their depressions. Knowing that they were capable of fighting their illnesses might have further enhanced their success. Blumenthal concludes: "Simply taking a pill is very passive. Patients who exercised may have felt a greater sense of mastery over their condition and gained a greater sense of accomplishment. They felt more self-confident and had better self-esteem because they were able to do it themselves, and attributed their improvement to their ability to exercise."[5]

As impressive as this result seems, the study could not completely determine if the results were simply a consequence of the social aspect of the workouts because the participants exercised together. During these sessions, everyday worries seemed to be forgotten, and people made small talk and laughed. Perhaps the new friendships and the collective experience were the main reasons for the improved mood.

In order to exclude this possibility, researchers at the Cooper Institute's Science Research Center in Golden, Colorado, initiated a further study.[6] They encouraged 80 men and women who were sedentary, depressive, and not on medication to participate in a sports program that lasted eight weeks, with three to five sessions per week. They either walked on a treadmill or pedaled on a stationary bike, and were alone (except for gruff assistants who checked on them to make sure nobody was secretly resting).

Half the participants tried an easy program and in one week burned just three kilocalories per pound of bodyweight. Though their symptoms improved, the effect was small and thus could have been a chance finding.

The members of the second group burned eight kilocalories per pound. This consumption corresponds to moderate exercise, like a brisk 30-minute walk on most days of the week. The symptoms in this group decreased by 47 percent, and in 42 percent of the patients the symptoms disappeared completely. This confirms that physical exercise is as effective as antidepressants and psychotherapy. Interestingly, it did not matter if the patients worked out for three or five days per week. Burning the recommended amount of kilocalories in a week is the main objective.

PLAYING AGAINST PANIC

Psychiatrists report regularly on patients and cases in which physical training was found to help people suffering from anxiety. Yet only a few trials have been initiated to look into this phenomenon. In one study, 46 individuals with claustrophobia, affective panic disorder, or both participated in a ten-week program and were asked to jog a distance of 3.1 to 3.7 miles on three or four days of the week. The patients of a second group were inactive and received either standard medication (the antidepressant clomipramine) or a placebo. Compared to the placebo, the medication significantly improved the symptoms. Exercise was also better than placebo, though not as effective as the medication.

In the treatment of alcoholics and drug addicts, moderate training programs are by now quite widespread in Germany, although there are few studies about whether this actually affects the addiction. On the contrary, members of soccer and handball clubs often consume amazing numbers of cigarettes as well as alcoholic beverages like beer and schnapps. It might shock American readers, but in lower-level German soccer leagues, it is not too uncommon for substitute players to smoke while watching their peers play. After the game, players and their families often gather and open a keg of beer. People with addiction problems might do better to avoid such crowds and pick up healthy ways of exercising like walking and jogging. Andreas Broocks of Helios Kliniken in Schwerin, Germany, is among the leaders in the field of sports therapy in psychiatry, and he concludes: "Regular endurance training substantially improves the self-confidence and self esteem of addicted patients and thus could help them to stay abstinent."[7]

Individuals with schizophrenia are also often in a condition for which physical exercise is much needed. Many such patients are heavy smokers, have an unhealthy diet, and hardly move their bodies. A training regimen would not only improve their physical shape but also help work against the psychiatric disorders that can accompany schizophrenia. According to one study, about 50 percent of all schizophrenic people also have symptoms of panic, obsessive-compulsive disorder, and depression. Although the possible benefit of exercise has not been studied until now, some physicians are discovering its potential. Inspired by good experiences with patients, many clinics are now trying to treat patients with schizophrenia with exercise as therapy.[8]

SOUND BODY FOR A SOUND MIND

It is thanks to the Roman poet Juvenal that we believe a sound mind (*mens sana*) resides in a sound body (*corpore sano*).[9] This proverb has spread for centuries, but it was not until recent times that neuroscientists have found enough evidence to reassure us that the ancient claim can be taken literally. Researchers have now accumulated evidence showing that exercise can stave off mental decline and the onset of widespread Alzheimer's disease, which leads to the loss of critical brain functions.

Alzheimer's is a disease that strikes with age. Among people aged 70 to 74, it is estimated that fewer than 3 percent are affected; among those older than 90, about one-third are affected. And because people in the United States and other industrialized nations live longer and longer, Alzheimer's is considered one of the most pressing health-care problems of the near future. An estimated 4.5 million Americans have Alzheimer's disease. That number has more than doubled since 1980 and is projected to reach 11.3 to 16 million by the year 2050.

Besides age, there are other risk factors. It may not be a good omen when family members have suffered from Alzheimer's because that suggests a genetic preposition to it. Alzheimer's also relatively frequently afflicts people with low education levels. These factors are hard to change once a person has reached adulthood, but there is another way to postpone the onset of the disease or to prevent it altogether: activities such as brisk walking or bicycle riding.

Results from lab trials indicate that exercise can protect the brain.[10] Mice held in cages with treadmills accumulate fewer harmful molecules in their brains than sedentary animals. These peptides, called amyloid beta, are usually found in demented mice and lead to plaque formation.

Even when this peptide is already spreading in the brain, exercise appears to help stall the progression of dementia. In a study published in the *Journal of Neuroscience*, researchers at the Institute for Brain Aging and Dementia at the University of California, Irvine, took mice that were predisposed to develop Alzheimer's disease and gave them running wheels for exercise. After several months of exercise, the mice showed improved cognitive behaviors and less amyloid-beta plaque. "What we found is that levels of the amyloid in these exercising mice went down," said the principal investigator, Carl Cotman. "Instead of a drug, it was a natural behavior that translated to a reduction of Alzheimer's-like pathology developing in the brain."[11]

A similar picture emerges when researchers try to correlate the lifestyles of people and their risk of developing Alzheimer's disease. Chinese researchers studied more than 1,000 elderly inhabitants of Beijing for three years. Those who hardly left their apartments developed dementia more often than was average.

Japanese researchers conducted a diligent study in which they monitored 828 citizens older than age 65 for seven years and inspected their brains using CT scans and other methods. More than 200 participants died in the course of the study, but most of their brains were examined after death. And the result showed again that sedentary seniors were more prone to become ill with Alzheimer's disease.[12]

Fortunately, there is no need for strenuous activities to stave off this notorious atrophy of the brain. Older men aged 71 to 93 who walk at least two miles every day cut the risk of Alzheimer's in half, compared to people the same age who walk only a quarter of a mile per day.[13]

The more intense the dose of exercise, the bigger the effect against dementia. This direct correlation was revealed by a five-year trial of elderly women. The most active women had a risk reduction by 50 percent, and a 60 percent reduction specifically for Alzheimer's.

One of the most extensive studies has been carried out by researchers at the Aging Research Center of the Karolinska Institute in Stockholm. In 1972 they began studying the leisure-time exercise habits of nearly 1,500 people.[14] Those who exercised at least two days per week during midlife lowered their risk of developing Alzheimer's by 50 percent.

For people around age 40, this implies that if they start now on moderate exercise programs, like bicycling and walking, they might be rewarded on some not-too-distant day. The neurologist Miia Kivipelto, senior author of the study, said: "These findings may have wide implications for preventive healthcare; if an individual adopts an active lifestyle in youth and at midlife, this may increase their probability of enjoying both physically and cognitively vital years later in life."

Apart from these epidemiological findings, brain-imaging studies also indicate that exercise influences the risk for Alzheimer's disease. These images show that physical activity slows down the type of brain atrophy that usually comes with age. Between our 30th and 90th birthdays, approximately 15 to 25 percent of the brain's gray matter is lost, and the areas in charge of learning and memorizing shrink the most.

The psychologist Arthur Kramer of the University of Illinois in Urbana-Champaign was able to demonstrate the presence of this atrophy when he looked at the brains of 55 healthy elderly persons, using magnetic resonance imaging (MRI). But Kramer also had good news, at least for those people who had always been active. They were not only in good shape, but on average their brain atrophy was not as pronounced as that in sedentary people. Furthermore, they had specifically retained structures in the lateral and frontal areas of the brain, which are most important for complex cognitive functions.

After this finding, Kramer and his colleagues wanted to check whether moderate exercise might even reverse the usual course of brain atrophy. Healthy but sedentary volunteers aged 60 to 79 participated in an aerobic training program for six months (consisting of one-hour sessions, three days per week). To provide a comparison, other volunteers of the same age also met three days per week in the gym. But instead of true exercising, they just did some stretching.

The astonishing result has been published in the *Journal of Gerontology*.[15] Parts of the brain actually increased in size for aerobic exercisers! The enlarged areas were primarily located in prefrontal and temporal cortices, the same regions often reported as showing substantial age-related deterioration. Declines in these areas are linked to a broad array of clinical symptoms including Alzheimer's disease. In the group that just did some stretching, such enlargements could not be found.

If this novel and intriguing finding is further confirmed, it will have profound repercussions for the prevention of neurodegenerative diseases. The results suggest that brain volume loss is not an inevitable effect of advancing age and that relatively minor interventions can halt or slow down this loss. Moderate exercise not only helps stave off the onset of cognitive decline, but it might have the potential to halt and even *reverse* the loss of brain structures in old age! These implications did not escape the attention of the researchers. They conclude that their results "directly bear on issues of public policy and clinical recommendations in that they suggest a rather simple and inexpensive mechanism to ward off the effects of senescence on human brain tissue."[16]

Responsible doctors are prudent enough not to raise hopes that Alzheimer's patients will have effective drugs available to them in the foreseeable future. At the same time, surveys show that more than 40 percent of adults who are 50 or older are afraid of losing control of their minds someday because of Alzheimer's disease. Science has rarely provided us with better arguments to start moving.

TRAINING IS THE BETTER PILL

As soon as we start sweating, we help our brains. As we saw, growth factors and neurotransmitters start circulating in higher numbers through the brain. Next, the number and length of connections between the nerve cells increase. One could say that the whole brain becomes jazzed up from inside, making it more malleable and more plastic than before. Yet there is an even more astonishing rejuvenator, which we will discuss in the following chapter; exercise appears to promote the growth of new nerve cells in old brains.

11

A Fountain of Youth in the Brain

EVERY DAY, THE NEUROSCIENTIST JEFFREY MACKLIS OFFERED HIS MICE
A new treat to sniff. One morning, he would blow the smell of
chocolate into their cage; the next, he would let them breathe
clouds of rosewater.

This way, Macklis introduced the mice to a previously unknown world. The animals were raised in scent-proof habitats
and had not experienced a single one of the dozen odors they
had been smelling in the course of his experiment. How
would their brains respond to novel stimuli?

Macklis and his colleagues at the Center for Nervous System Repair at Massachusetts General Hospital and Harvard
Medical School in Boston were the first researchers to see
what happens in the part of the brain where odors are
processed. They achieved this feat by following the fate of new
nerve cells that migrate to the olfactory bulb, the brain region
enabling us to sense smells. There, new nerve cells appear to
originate all the time. But only when animals smell a previously unknown scent do these nascent nerve cells mature into
active neurons that integrate themselves into the brain's circuits two to three weeks later. The nerve cells develop long

axons and make numerous connections—synapses—to other neurons. In contrast to these new arrivals, the older neurons that form the existing network within the olfactory bulb barely get excited by a new odor. "The new neurons are not replacing the old ones," says Macklis. "They have a unique function: learn new smells."[1]

New nerve cells for new memories: Elkhonon Goldberg, a clinical psychologist at New York University, believes in this formula, too. Time and again, in his office, two blocks south of Central Park, elderly individuals show up who often misplace their keys, leave the stove burning, or forget what is on the pages of the books they have just read.

To combat their forgetfulness, Goldberg prescribes a program intended to improve several cognitive functions, such as vocabulary retention, mental agility, and spatial perception. To create this program, the psychologist analyzed 200 tests used for the treatment of stroke patients and combined the elements of nearly 60 of them. Two days per week, he requires patients to solve problems presented on a computer screen. A typical task during one such hour-long session is to determine the pattern underlying an arrangement of colored triangles, squares, and circles.

Each individual program usually runs for three months, and at the end Goldberg assesses whether the sessions have improved his patients' memories in everyday life. After the first 100 patients who tried this course, says Goldberg, he was "pleasantly impressed." In around 60 percent of the cases, incremental memory loss had been stopped; in 30 percent, the patients' power to recall things had actually improved.

"Our successes are probably due to the growth of fresh nerve cells in the brain," says Goldberg. "Cognitive activities can trigger the birth of new neurons."[2]

NEUROGENESIS: NEW NERVE CELLS IN THE BRAIN

A fountain of youth in the brain? New mental power thanks to new nerve cells? Until recently, Macklis and Goldberg would have been dismissed as dreamers because they call into question a seemingly irrefutable dogma: our nerve cells lose their power to divide shortly after we are born. If so, the human brain could at best keep its established level of mental capacity, which in most cases would shrink with age.

But these days, neurologists, biochemists, and physicians see more and more data indicating otherwise: new nerve cells do grow in certain parts of the adult brain. With awe and surprise, researchers realize this process—called neurogenesis—appears to be essential for the normal functioning of the brain.

"We are beginning to see the brain from a completely different perspective," says Gerd Kempermann, a leading expert on neurogenesis now at the Center for Regenerative Therapies in Dresden.[3] "There is a positive tendency: The development of the brains goes on during the whole life."

It is especially encouraging that new nerve cells sprouting in old brains turn out to be particularly malleable and flexible. For that reason, they seem to contribute to the astonishing reserve capacities that allow the brain to master difficult and unexpected challenges. Kempermann says: "The neurogenesis is probably a fundamental precondition for staying mentally alert up to high age."

The emerging picture of neurogenesis implies that genetics alone do not determine whether people retain mental acuity throughout their lives. Rather, lifestyle—the way we treat the brain—has tremendous repercussions on its ability to renew itself. And, among these ways, it's physical exercise that appears most important because it promotes the production of fresh nerve cells.

The effect of neurogenesis on exercise is apparently due to an ancient mechanism shaped by evolution: the more an animal moves around in its environment, the greater the likelihood that it will encounter novel situations. Thus, the brain of an active creature produces especially high numbers of nerve cells that can be used to process these new stimuli. The new cells mature into fully functioning neurons when they are challenged with new tasks. In the absence of such challenges, it is thought, a big portion of the new nerve cells die before long. And in the absence of physical activity, the production of new nerve cells largely ceases.

It's not easy to prove that neurogenesis takes place in the adult brains of humans. Nearly all of the relevant data stem from animal studies because, for obvious reasons, scientists cannot perform crucial experiments on humans (such as tracing radioactive bits of DNA in neural networks) to see if nerve cells are new. However, a growing body of indirect evidence leaves no doubt neurogenesis takes place in the human brain. American scientists have published an especially convincing study. They encouraged 11 healthy women and men to train for three months in the gym at Columbia University in New York and thereafter analyzed their brains by magnetic resonance imaging (MRI). In the course of the workouts, a particular area within the hippocampus became increasingly supplied with blood. Parallel studies on mice by the same scientists revealed what this means: new capillaries as well as new nerve cells grow there.[4]

Fred Gage, of the Salk Institute in La Jolla, California, was among the researchers who carried out this study. He and his co-workers Gerd Kempermann and Henriette van Praag first showed that physical exercise can literally act as a fertilizer for the brain. They discovered this by keeping mice in cages with running wheels, so the animals could run as much as they liked. The mobilized mice produced an above-average number of new nerve cells, compared to mice kept without the wheels.[5] The effect was actually so big that, ever since Gage's findings were published, researchers studying neurogenesis also keep their mice in environments allowing them to move. Only under these circumstances do the mice produce fresh neurons in numbers large enough to be studied.

However, does this supply of fresh nerve cells actually make the mice smarter? This is what Henriette van Praag, then a senior researcher in the Gage lab, was able to prove.[6] Her experiments actually started when a small biotech company in La Jolla went out of business. The firm had lab mice left over and asked van Praag if she might need some. She happily accepted the offer because these mice were exactly the kind she had been looking for. The animals were 19 months old (equaling a human age of 60), and they had been kept all their lives in small and narrow cages. Thus they were ideal for studying the impact of exercise on old, dulled brains.

Van Praag put half of these mice into cages equipped with running wheels, where the rodents usually ran more than three miles per day. The other half were still kept in cages without the benefit of exercise. After 35 days, van Praag tested the memories of all the mice by putting them into a special water maze. It consisted of a small pool with a shallow platform in the middle, just under the surface. Because mice dislike swimming, they stay on the platform whenever possible, and when repeatedly dropped into the water, will eventually memorize the platform's location and swim to it.

It turned out that the performance of mice in this environment correlated to the amount of exercise they had been granted. "The aged and sedentary mice just swam around and gave up. Many of them floated and waited for me to take them out of the pool," Praag recalls. Whereas it took these sedentary animals an average of 30 seconds to find the platform, the physically fit mice needed only 15 seconds to get there.

But was this enhanced learning really due to the production of new nerve cells? To find an answer, the mice were sacrificed and their brains studied 10 days after the test to determine the number of new nerve cells in their brains. Indeed, the mice that had been allowed to run in their cages, and had performed well in the test, had significantly more new neurons in the hippocampus. The brains of these aged runners, who had formerly been kept for so long in narrow cages, had been rejuvenated by exercise.[7]

Henriette van Praag is convinced that elderly people can benefit greatly from physical exercise. She believes it is worthwhile to "buy your aging relatives a treadmill." Fred Gage has a similar take on this himself and exercises regularly (he plays squash, runs, and does light weightlifting). The slim and energetic neuroscientist has changed how people see the brain. When I visited him in his lab, he told me: "Your brain is not a computer but a plastic organ—and the way it changes can be controlled by you."

The discovery of neurogenesis not only changes our perception of the healthy brain but also alters our understanding of why and how brains develop certain illnesses. Alzheimer's disease, which leads to the loss of many mental functions, and the movement disorder Parkinson's disease, were until recently usually ascribed to the loss and death of nerve tissue. Now, physicians are starting to rethink matters and view things from a different perspective. Are these untreatable diseases triggered because the production of new nerve cells is stalling?

Also, for learning disorders, depression, alcoholism, nicotine addiction, and schizophrenia, researchers increasingly discuss whether a lack of neurogenesis might play a role— and what sort of activity, including physical exercise, appears to help against precisely these diseases. The scientific exploration of neurogenesis "has evolved into one of the most interesting and most promising projects of modern neuroscience and in particular of molecular psychiatry," concludes Amelia Eisch of the University of Texas's Southwestern Medical Center in Dallas.[8]

Yet some findings remain mysterious. Why is it, for example, that the capability to grow new nerve cells is restricted only to a part of the forebrain and the dentate gyrus of the hippocampus, an area important for learning and memory? This limitation seems even stranger because most other parts of the brain have progenitor cells and stem cells, which have the biological potential of maturing into fully functional neurons. But instead of doing this, they lie dormant, the sleeping beauties of the brain.

To awaken these cells and make them grow is a dream of medicine already pursued by many pharmaceutical companies as well as academic researchers. Brain, the motto goes, heal thyself!

THE MYTH OF THE STATIC BRAIN

This hope and excitement centers on a phenomenon that was doubted and dismissed by almost all neuroscientists in the last century. They were under the influence of a verdict by the famous Spanish brain researcher and Nobel laureate, Santiago Ramón y Cajal. In 1928, he famously declared: "In adult centers the nerve paths are something fixed, ended, immutable. Everything may die, nothing may regenerate."

A few scientists dared to question this verdict but were not taken seriously and were even ridiculed. One of these skeptics was Joseph Altman, who carried out fascinating experiments at the Massachusetts Institute of Technology (MIT) in the 1960s. He fed food that contained low-level radioactive chemicals needed to make DNA to rats, cats, and guinea pigs. If the animals produced new nerve cells, they would incorporate the radioactive labeled chemicals into the nuclei of these new cells. And indeed, Altman was able to detect radioactive signals in the brain tissue after he killed the animals and performed autopsies on them—a sure sign that neurogenesis had occurred. In hindsight, it seems odd, but other researchers simply ignored Altman's findings. This neglect harmed Altman's career; he was forced to leave MIT and take a position at a less well-known school.

Ten years later, the researcher Michael Kaplan of the University of New Mexico took pictures with an electron microscope showing newly grown neurons. But he was ignored and ridiculed as well. Kaplan once recounted how the influential neuroscientist Pasko Rakic of Yale University dismissed his results: "Those may look like neurons in New Mexico. But they don't in New Haven."[9]

Rakic even came up with a theory why neurons in the adult brain were unable to divide: at one point during evolution, our forebears had traded the capability of producing new nerve cells for the ability to store memories in a constant number of nerve cells. For reasons of stability, Rakic believed, there was simply no space reserved for new neurons in the human brain.

Eventually, singing canaries greatly contributed to overturning the old, false dogma of the static brain. The male birds sing their songs in the spring, but over the summer lose their repertoire like feathers in the molt—only to impress female birds the next spring with a completely new set of melodies.

One day, as he was taking a shower, it occurred to the biologist Fernando Nottebohm of Rockefeller University in New York how the male canaries accomplish this trick: the areas of the brain containing the memories of the old melodies die off and are replaced by new neurons the next spring. Experiments using radioactive DNA have confirmed Nottebohm's hunch: male canaries indeed produce thousands of new nerve cells per day.

Initially, it was believed that only birds were capable of re-growing brain tissue. But when scientists looked into other species, they found neurogenesis all over the place: frogs, lizards, rodents, and monkeys do it. Why, then, should humans be an exception?

It took quite a while to come up with the ultimate proof. But in 1998, Swedish and American brain researchers realized there was a way to see if neurogenesis takes place in the adult human brain. Physicians routinely inject radioactive, labeled DNA building blocks into severely ill cancer patients. By doing so, they are trying to find out how many new cancer cells grow in a patient's tumors. However, because the labeled DNA is incorporated into any type of dividing cells, new nerve cells should be detectable, too. The researchers were granted permission to study five patients with advanced cancer of the larynx. After their deaths, the patients' brain tissue was analyzed. The result? Until the last days of their lives, these people had produced new neurons in their brains.

Since this milestone discovery, researchers agree that an adult produces thousands of neurons in the hippocampus every day. In comparison to the roughly 100 billion neurons that comprise the brain, this might appear a small amount. However, the new neurons possess a juvenile excitability lost by the old neurons. The neuroscientist Gerd Kempermann is convinced they have an important impact on our mental capabilities: "Apparently a rather small number of newly produced cells is sufficient to profoundly alter the network architecture of our brain."[10]

It is evident that freshly produced neurons greatly contribute to a phenomenon called neuroplasticity, the brain's surprising capability to adapt to a constantly changing environment. At least three different mechanisms contribute to the plasticity of the brain. First, existing connections between nerve cells, the synapses, can be strengthened within seconds, allowing us to remember what we just heard, felt, or thought. Second, as new synapses sprout, they create a dynamic neuronal network that can store memories for long periods of time. Finally, the production of new nerve cells—a process that takes many days—can bring enduring changes upon the brain. Many studies have added weight to the belief that neurogenesis is an "important part of plasticity," says Amelia Eisch of the University of Texas Southwestern Medical Center in Dallas.[11]

In short: a few extremely versatile neurons are pivotal for the brain's lifelong ability to change itself. Like a muscle that grows when used, the cells of the gray matter thrive when challenged. New neurons in the olfactory bulb develop when they encounter odors, and new neurons in the hippocampus mature when they receive input worth remembering.

BRAIN FITNESS

The phenomenon of neurogenesis could actually be the long-sought mechanism by which the environment is able to shape and put its imprint upon the brain. Many empirical studies have shown how important physical activity is among these environmental influences. Both physical and cognitive exercises appear to prevent or delay degenerative processes in the aging brain. Researchers at Rush Presbyterian-St. Luke's Medical Center in Chicago carried out a study of 642 elderly people with varying educational backgrounds. It turned out that with each additional year of formal education, the risk of developing Alzheimer's disease was reduced by 17 percent; several other studies also suggest that a good education can stave off the onset of Alzheimer's.

In the late 1980s Robert Katzman of the University of California in San Diego studied this effect in more detail. In his view, learning and studying increases the density of the synapses in the brain—thereby enhancing something called "cognitive reserve." The bigger the cognitive reserve, reasoned Katzman, the better the brain can cope with the loss of nerve cells due to illness and age.[12]

This concept was supported by a study of 130 Catholic priests and nuns. During their lives, their cognitive capabilities were assessed. After their natural deaths, autopsies on their brains were performed. Plaques (protein deposits that interfere with neural networks) typical of Alzheimer's disease were found in all brains with the same frequency, regardless of the level of education each had received. It turned out, however, that these plaques affected the brains in varying degrees. Those people with an extensive education had retained their cognitive capabilities much better than people with less education. The differences were profound: better-educated individuals started to show symptoms of Alzheimer's only when they had five times as many plaques in their brains as people with lower levels of education. The former group possessed a substantial cognitive reserve enabling them to compensate for the effects of Alzheimer's.

Your current occupation—reading—as well as playing cards, or doing crafts, can help preserve the cognitive functions, believes the neurologist Robert Friedland at the Case Western Reserve University in Cleveland: "I believe they all involve learning in some way."[13] That would mean an interesting job keeps one healthy, whereas retiring early in life might be a fatal step toward dulling the mind.

In any case, watching television should be avoided. According to Friedland's research, gawking at the screen increases the risk of being afflicted with Alzheimer's disease. He and his colleagues asked the partners and relatives of 135 Alzheimer patients about their activities before the onset of the disease.[14] Subsequently, they compared these data with answers from 331 healthy people. The study results reveal that the Alzheimer's patients spent a much larger part of their lives in front of the television set than healthy people. With each hour of watching television per day, the risk of Alzheimer's increased by a factor of 1.3. That does not necessarily mean the content of television programs dulls the mind (though there is no shortage of stupid shows), but rather frequent television consumption might point toward a lifestyle lacking both physical and mental activity. "Time spent on television viewing may reflect a desire to avoid more stimulating activities and may be indicative of a mentally inactive lifestyle which has been shown to be associated with increased risk of cognitive decline with age," the authors conclude.[15]

Conversely, an active lifestyle turns out to be an effective remedy against this cognitive decline experienced by so many elderly people. Ulman Lindenberger and Martin Lövdén at the Max Planck Institute for Human Development in Berlin have followed 516 persons at ages 70 to 100 and recorded the degree of their "social participation."[16] In interviews they asked specific questions about their daily lives: Did they have company the day prior to the interview? Have they recently been involved in hobbies? How often did they dine out, and did they still go to social events like concerts? The data covered a period of eight years and revealed that activity, possibly by triggering beneficial neurological processes, can protect the brain. People who led an active and engaged life showed a significantly smaller cognitive decline than people with limited social participation. An active lifestyle after retirement can mean many different things: music, sports, strenuous playing with grandchildren, studying a language, political activism, hiking, or writing a book. These and other similar activities can serve to keep the brain young.

Physical exercise further enhances this effect. Lindenberger explains this using the example of crossing a street on foot: usually, this task would be more demanding for the brain of an 80-year-old person than for the brain of a teenager. However, if an old person keeps his body in good shape by regular exercising, the attention needed for the motor task of crossing the street is minimal. "Thus, mental energy is saved and can be utilized for other purely cognitive activities," Lindenberger explains. His example shows how the model of "cognitive reserve" must be expanded. Not only mental activities, but also physical activities, contribute to the resilience of the brain.

12

Cancer: A Growing Case for Exercise

ABOUT 50 EPIDEMIOLOGICAL STUDIES HAVE SHOWN THAT PHYSICAL exercise reduces the risk for colon cancer. In a scientific first, researchers at the Fred Hutchinson Cancer Research Center in Seattle were able to demonstrate this protection on the level of individual cells. Their study included 102 healthy men, who were divided into two groups. Half the participants were asked to conduct one hour of aerobic activity per day (six days a week); the other half carried on with life as usual. After one year, the doctors took colon tissue samples, biopsies, and examined them under the microscope. That way, they were able to detect how many of the colon cells were about to divide. A jump in cell division can be a warning sign of cancer.

The analysis revealed that there were fewer actively dividing cells in men who exercised diligently for an average of four hours of activity per week. Those with more than five hours of weekly exercise demonstrated an even smaller rate of proliferation. The other half of the men, who hardly exercised at all, did not have the beneficial effect.[1]

Besides colon cancer, breast cancer can be prevented by physical activity. Even when women become active after entering menopause, they lower their breast cancer risk by 20 percent. To see this effect, it is sufficient to be active for 30 minutes for five days per week, doing things like brisk walking or bicycling. The advantages were biggest for slim and slightly overweight women. Though obese women did not profit, they, too, can reap the benefit by reducing their weight to normal and making themselves more likely to realize the preventive effect.

One large study in Europe has even revealed that chores and housework, such as vacuuming, cooking, washing, ironing, and housecleaning, can help stave off cancer. The researchers assessed the activity levels and the health status of 218,169 women for more than six years. Active women spent an average of 16 to 17 hours a week on household chores— and had a reduced breast cancer risk of 20 percent (younger women) to 30 percent (menopausal women) compared to inactive controls. The researchers are not saying that women should be stay-at-home mothers doing all the chores. Rather, the study reiterates a message that is true for both genders: the benefits of exercise kick in at relatively low intensities.[2]

Finally, the risk for prostate cancer is also reduced by physical exercise. In the United States it is one the most prevalent cancers among men, whereas it is far rarer among men living in Asian countries. However, as men from Japan or China immigrate to the United States and adopt the Western lifestyle, their prostate cancer risk approaches that of American men. Apart from diet, lack of exercise plays a major role influencing the risk for prostate cancer by 10 to 70 percent.

But how can an active life stave off cancer? As with colon cancer, there appears to be a link to digestion. In sedentary bodies the peristalsis of the colon is slowed down. Thus, cancer-causing agents in the food stay for an extended time in the colon. The researchers have also identified numerous other factors that help to prevent tumor growth.[3]

BODY FAT AND DANGEROUS HORMONE LEVELS

Physical activity reduces weight and thus the production of female sex hormones, especially estrogens because these are made not only in the ovaries but also in the fat tissue. That is why lack of exercise often leads to both fat deposits and elevated hormone levels, which can promote the growth of tumors in the cervix, endometrium, ovaries, and breast.

The most natural way to reduce the level of these hormones is physical activity. Anne McTiernan of the Fred Hutchinson Cancer Research Center has demonstrated this in a trial of 267 women who did not take artificial hormones.[4] Researchers weighed the women, noted their weekly amount of exercise, and assessed their levels of the hormones estradiol and estrone. These hormones are very active and can promote breast cancer.

The result: women who are heavy and hardly move have hormone levels exceeding those of active and normal-weight women by 50 to 100 percent. So by watching their weight and performing some moderate exercise, women can reduce hormone levels under their own steam to a "healthy level," concludes McTiernan.[5]

According to her study, 30 minutes of moderate training, five days per week, is sufficient. The exercise appears to increase the level of certain proteins that in turn can remove excess hormone levels from the blood.[6] Furthermore, it beneficially influences the pathways that are involved in the production of hormones. In physically fit bodies there is a high level of certain intermediate products that cannot be converted into hormones. By comparison, in overweight women there is a high level of products than can be turned into hormones. In addition, exercise seems to be connected with an advantageous composition of the breast tissue. A trial in Norway showed that women who get at least two hours of activity per week have less dense breast tissue than sedentary women. And the higher the tissue density, the higher the breast cancer risk.[7]

The cancer-causing potential of these hormones is widely known and acknowledged in medical research. All the more odd, then, that pharmaceutical companies manufacture estrogen products and still, despite large studies showing risk, sell them as "hormone replacement therapy" (HRT) to menopausal women. In the United States, a large trial of 16,000 women had to be terminated as the emerging data from it revealed that the hormone products do more harm than good: If 10,000 women take the products estrogen and progestogen for one year, eight more of them will develop breast cancer than those who do not take them. Even though these pills were also touted as preventive against heart disease, they were also cardiovascular dangers. What miserable credentials for a product that is claimed to be a remedy.[8]

Women who take hormone pills face a higher risk of cancer, for two possible reasons. As mentioned, estrogens can trigger the growth of cells in the breast tissue. Moreover, hormone consumption affects behavior and dampens the desire to exercise. Studies with mice suggest a direct link. The more estrogens given to female mice, the less distance they ran on a treadmill.[9] Because of the wide publicity given the large trial that had to be stopped, many fewer women are taking pills. Many of the benefits supposedly offered by the replacement hormones, such as a more youthful appearance or a healthier heart, are more easily found on a hike or at a gym.

EXERCISE AS CANCER PREVENTION

People who exercise also influence their immune system, and thereby their cancer risk. But the effect of exercise can go both ways. An overload can weaken the immune system and even promote the growth of a tumor. On the other hand, the right dose of exercise does strengthen the immune system and can hinder or inhibit tumor growth. Moderate exercise appears to promote the production of certain cells of the immune system. Cytotoxic T cells, natural killer cells, and similar cells patrol the body and are capable of destroying tumor cells. The members of the beneficial platoon of cells have been shown to be produced in bigger numbers by "regular, moderate exercise."[10] Mice allowed to run as much as they want, on running wheels, boost their production of natural killer cells. They then have significant advantages compared to sedentary mice because their immune systems can fight more cancer cells, and fewer tumors grow.

With age, the immune system becomes weaker, and physicians suspect this decline is one of the reasons cancer risk increases with age. The aging process can be clearly seen in T cells. Their number dwindles in the course of the years, and their ability to detect and fight foreign cells becomes weaker. However, this decline can be halted and reversed: Elderly women and men were shown to improve the function of their T cells by exercise compared with sedentary controls of the same age.[11] This finding points to an additional mechanism that underlies the cancer-fighting potential of exercise: it counteracts the age-related decline of the immune system.

Another support for the cancer-preventing effects of exercise can be found in studies of diabetes. Insulin produced in the pancreas is needed by cells so that they can absorb glucose from the blood and store it. The level of insulin must correspond to the body's needs, and if this balance is destroyed, the likelihood for developing cancer increases.

Patients suffering from type 2 diabetes have been found to produce higher quantities of a protein called insulin-like growth factor I (IGF-I), which is thought to trigger cancerous growth. The rates of colon, liver, pancreas, endometrium, and breast cancer are in fact higher among people with type 2 diabetes.[12] That does not sound good at all, but luckily one can do something about it: Physical exercise, as we saw, can reverse the symptoms of diabetes and also appears to lower the IGF-I level.

BMI AND CANCER

As they continue to explore the causes of cancer, doctors ascribe a greater role to obesity than they once did. British scientists reviewing data pooled from more than 140 studies have just confirmed that the risk of developing a number of common and some less common cancers goes up with increasing BMI.[13] An earlier study had already revealed that the risk of obese men for developing an extraordinarily aggressive version of prostate cancer is increased by 80 percent.[14] Thomas Hawighorst and Günter Emons, at the University Hospital Göttingen, Germany, published a review article on the subject painting a very somber but realistic picture. By now, there is "sufficiently hard evidence for the connection between adiposity and an elevated risk for cancer" of the endometrium, the kidney, the breast, the colon, and esophagus, whereas, "The prognosis for adipose women with breast cancer is worse, and gaining weight after the diagnosis also has a bad prognostic effect."[15]

The American Cancer Society published a particularly extensive survey on the subject.[16] The study started more than 20 years ago and included more than 900,000 women and men. Their average age was 57, and none had any tumor-based diseases. In the following 16 years, 6.3 percent of them died because of a condition that was caused by cancer. Then, the researchers analyzed the data to see whether there was a link between the death rate and body weight. In order not to distort their findings, they excluded risk factors and used only data from people who never had smoked.

According to the study, the risk for dying from cancer is approximately 10 percent higher for women with a BMI between 25 and 29.9 and three times higher for women with a BMI between 30 to 40. And extremely obese women have a risk for dying from cancer that is elevated by 88 percent, compared to normal-weight women. The data of the men revealed a similarly gloomy picture.

In total, the researchers figure that obesity causes about 20 percent of all deaths of women related to cancer. Among men, the number is about 14 percent. The experts of the International Agency for Research on Cancer in Lyon, France, estimate that 25 percent of cancer cases worldwide are caused by excess weight or obesity and a sedentary lifestyle.[17]

Apart from overeating, lack of exercise is in most cases the reason why people balloon and develop a pathological condition. Excess fat on the body impairs the whole metabolism and causes several of the risks mentioned earlier. The biochemistry of the estrogens becomes messed up, and the insulin system gets out of balance. The longer an affected person remains physically inactive, the worse everything gets—because muscle mass is incrementally replaced with fat.

Love handles and potbellies are by no means passive additions to a body; rather, they actively interfere with some processes in the rest of the organism. Certain messenger substances, so called adipocytokines, are produced by fat tissue and can play a role in the development of cancer. The experts Hawighorst and Emons conclude that in obese people "the metabolic-biochemical effects of overweight can cause the formation of a malignant tumor in a multi-level process."[18]

Researchers still speculate whether and if exercise affects an already existing tumor. Physical activity increases the demand for oxygen and nutrients—which might starve the tumor of these resources. If the blood is primarily pumped into the muscles, one could reason that there is not much left to feed the tumor.

Although evidence continues to accumulate that being physically active reduces a person's risk for developing certain cancers, to date, the many details of the mechanism remain unknown. Many factors may act together and might vary from individual to individual. However, even though the ideal amount of exercise to prevent cancer has yet to be determined, doctors and physiologists working in the field are convinced that becoming active is worthwhile anyhow. As Kim Westerlind of the AMC Cancer Research Center in Denver, Colorado, concludes, "It would appear reasonable to suggest that regular moderate physical activity be incorporated into [a] healthy lifestyle for all its already well-established benefits, as well as to potentially reduce cancer risk."[19]

EXERCISE AND QUALITY OF LIFE IN CANCER PATIENTS

The doctrines of few medical fields have been as drastically turned around as they have in cancer medicine. Generations of doctors had been taught that people diagnosed with cancer primarily needed rest. Patients were discouraged from exercising, out of the erroneous belief that this would worsen their health. When the physician Klaus Schüle established the world's first training group for cancer patients in Cologne, Germany, many of his colleagues were outraged. A radiologist warned him: "Can you guarantee you are not going to trigger metastases?" Schüle replied: "Can you guarantee that your rays don't trigger growth of new tumors?"[20]

By rejecting exercise for their cancer patients, medical doctors did more harm than good, says Fernando Dimeo of the Hospital Charité in Berlin. "During chemotherapy and the weeks and months to follow patients were put in a passive role. Doctors were afraid of overburdening them and advised many of the patients not to participate in sports and demanding activity even in the long term."[21]

But recommending cancer patients to take it easy has severe consequences. At first, people are shocked to learn they have cancer. Then, they are told not to use their bodies much any longer—which makes the situation even more devastating because they now feel completely at the mercy of their illness. On top of this, being confined to rest worsens the impact of chemotherapy and of the cancer drugs, which can cause anemia and heart problems and loss of strength as well as vitality. As a result they are tired, and they become short of breath. "These symptoms can be worsened by lack of exercise and the subsequent loss of endurance," warns Dimeo.

In no time the patient is caught in a vicious circle of declining activity and decreasing resilience. Recovery is slowed after each stage of cancer treatment, thereby causing even more inactivity. After a while, a patient enters a phase regarded as a disease in its own right, the so-called fatigue syndrome. Once the cancer treatment is completed, this condition is the biggest problem many patients face—and can be a direct consequence of medically prescribed lack of exercise.

Too much rest can also worsen the primary disease. As we saw, women diagnosed with cancer have a worse prognosis when they put on five kilograms or more during their cancer treatments. Intriguingly, many patients themselves have intuitively sensed that rest was not good at all for them—and decided to do something about it. In the United States many people diagnosed with cancer began exercising hard because they hoped this might improve their quality of life and survival chances. One of the pioneers of this movement is Anna Schwartz. When she fell sick with non-Hodgkin's lymphoma, she reminded herself of what had often struck her when she worked as a nurse in an oncology clinic. Those patients who, despite the exhausting treatment, regularly left their rooms and stayed physically active "were in a better mood," Schwartz recalls. And when she had to go through chemotherapy, she forced herself to exercise. She went jogging and played tennis—despite a catheter for the cancer drugs in her body.

Since then, this thoroughly fit woman, who is considered as good as cured, has turned her story into a job. Research grants from the National Institutes of Health enabled her to carry out scientific studies on the subject. In the resulting publications Schwartz has shown that exercise indeed ameliorates the fatigue syndrome and makes patients stronger again.[22]

Since then, Schwartz has been offering horse riding for cancer patients in Cave Creek, Arizona, has been giving talks, and has written a book about fitness and cancer.[23] The preface was penned by Lance Armstrong who, after overcoming testicular cancer, won the Tour de France seven times. Armstrong himself has declared that he was better and stronger after his illness than before. "When people are diagnosed, their first impression is 'Oh my god, I am going to die,'" he once said. "Over time, they lose that impression. They get the confidence back, they know they are going to live, they get back to life, they get back to work and they get back to exercise."[24]

Encouraged by Armstrong's incredible story, cancer patients began improving their odds and their lives by exercising—although many oncologists still dismissed sports, thinking its strain and stress would only weaken patients' immune systems. By now, however, this patients' movement has led to a change of thinking among many doctors, says Julia Rowland of the National Cancer Institute in Bethesda, Maryland. Many new studies have been initiated to reveal the impact of exercise on cancer patients.

The results, says Rowland, have shown that the oncologists' worries have been unfounded. In many cases exercise actually does improve the mood of the patients and their strength, while lowering the side effects of radiation and chemotherapy.[25] When breast cancer patients try strength training two days per week, both physical and mental strength improve significantly.[26]

Yet exercise does not need to be a daunting activity or even an organized outing to produce significant rewards for breast cancer survivors, researchers at the University of Texas M. D. Anderson Cancer Center, in Houston, have found. Over the course of six months, they regularly met with women who had gone through breast cancer treatment and led sedentary lives. At the meetings the women were encouraged to integrate physical activities like brisk walking and climbing stairs into their lives, five days per week, at least 30 minutes at a time.

After six months, the mobilized women showed many improvements. In contrast with inactive patients, they felt much healthier and had less pain and fewer handicaps. Their constitutions were substantially strengthened, which was documented by a small competition at the end of the study: the active women were able to walk faster than the inactive ones. "The wonderful take-away message from this study is that simple exercises, such as walking during coffee breaks or parking farther away from work, can have beneficial effects on physical health and functioning," says the study's principal investigator, Karen Basen-Engquist.[27]

By now, some doctors prescribe exercise even when chemotherapy is still under way or right afterward. Most patients, it is true, do not feel like working out at all. Chemotherapy and radiation therapy not only destroy cancer cells, but also kill stem cells, which give rise, among other things, to cells of the immune system. Thus, immediately after treatment patients have few bodily defenses and are isolated in separate rooms to protect them from potentially deadly viruses and bacteria.

However, this well-intentioned isolation comes with a price, says the sports physician Klaus Schüle. In his pioneering work, he has found that bed rest significantly lowered the physical resilience of these individuals. The more rounds of cancer treatment they receive, the harder it is for them to recover. To change that, Schüle and three colleagues did something unheard of: they placed stationary bikes in the rooms of 32 patients and encouraged them to pedal for 10 to 20 minutes once or twice a day. Unlike 32 patients that had been isolated the old, sedentary way, these exercising patients recovered faster and more thoroughly from the side effects of cancer treatment. Even very sick patients actually do profit from exercise. They gain muscle strength and endurance without worsening the primary disease.[28]

EXERCISE AND SURVIVAL

Even the most optimistic physicians never seriously expected that physical exercise might prolong the life of cancer patients.

But in recent years data have started to emerge indicating that exercise indeed improves survival rates. The effects seen so far are modest in absolute numbers but relate to two of the most widespread and dangerous cancers. Two of the trials involve patients with colon cancer. One included 823 patients with early-stage or slightly advanced tumors that had surgery and adjuvant chemotherapy.[29] Six months after the completion of the therapy, Jeffrey Meyerhardt at Dana-Farber Cancer Institute in Boston asked them to report how much physical activity they had engaged in. The data show that exercise corresponding to walking for 60 minutes, six days per week "appears to reduce the risk of cancer recurrence and mortality."

Meyerhardt has produced similar results in another study in which he and his colleagues observed 573 women who had been treated for colon cancer.[30] Patients who started exercising after their diagnosis lived longer than sedentary ones; the survival rate was increased by 50 percent. Since that study, Jeffrey Meyerhardt tells his patients that "exercise might be advantageous for them."

Finally, the epidemiologist Michelle Holmes of Brigham & Women's Hospital in Boston has found a similar effect for breast cancer.[31] She and her colleagues analyzed the cancer progressions of nearly 3,000 women and found a significant correlation between the level of activity and survival. If a woman walks three to four hours per week, the risk of breast cancer death is lowered by 50 percent.

When an effect in a similar range is seen using a conventional cancer drug, leading doctors are quick to talk about a "major advance" or a "major turning point."[32] Meyerhardt and Holmes are much more cautious and say that their findings are not proof at this point. A correlation between cancer survival and exercise level does not prove that exercise was the cause. There is no study yet that would say a person can literally run away from cancer. However, more and more data point to the benefits of physical activity.

Now, many oncologists are eager to explore the cancer-fighting properties of exercise further and to carry out more studies. Which kind of exercise would be the best? What would be the ideal amount? However, will the drug industry fund such research? "There is no doubt that the pharmaceutical industry would back an agent with potential to reduce cancer recurrence by at least 50 percent," says Wendy Demark-Wahnefried of Duke University Medical Center in North Carolina. "But who will back a trial that evaluates the potential benefit of sneakers and sweatpants?"[33]

13

Longevity, Potency, and Resilience

AT AGE 20 THE IDEA OF GROWING OLD IS SOMETHING TO THINK about later in life. The body is still going strong; injuries and wounds and broken bones heal rapidly, and there is no moaning and groaning to be heard first thing in the morning. At age 40 wrinkles and the first aging marks appear and love handles may have established themselves in the midsection, but there is still no time to think about getting old. At age 60, people may have gone through one or two operations, perhaps after an unfortunate fall while on vacation. Among friends and acquaintances, the first deaths occur. Subtly one starts to get accustomed to the fact that the body may not be in the best shape. Hearts may start to beat out of rhythm, legs may be swollen in the evening, sleep is no longer so predictable.

This scenario is true for many people—but not for everyone. Around us are people who hardly seem to age, who look nearly the same in the course of many years. In the science department of my magazine there is a slim female colleague who, in the ten years I've known her, has never really changed. People guess that her age is about 48, but she is 61. Not long ago, such a woman would have been marveled at. In 1900, life expectancy at birth in the United States was 47 years,[1] but now it is 78 years at birth for the total population in the United States.[2] This increase in life span is remarkable—and unevenly distributed among the people. One person struggles with bad health and dies at age 60, while another lives to be 100. Why is it that some people's bodies break down, while others remain radiant with health?

When you pose this question to people who are blessed with long and healthy lives, it's striking to see how frequently they mention physical activity. On a campground in Sequoia National Park, in the Sierra Nevada Mountains in California, I met an 83-year-old man, Alan Buckley, and asked him about his secret as we held sticks with marshmallows into the fire. Even though many men of his age live in old people's homes, Buckley camps every summer in the mountains and looks in the evenings at the Milky Way before going to bed. So what is his secret? Buckley says he simply always walks when he moves around on his walnut tree plantation. He shakes his head when he thinks about the "weekend warriors," as he calls them, who sit in their cars and offices and armchairs during the week and try to make up for the missed exercise on the weekend.

Antonio Pierro also was always in motion. He was born in 1896 in Forenza, Italy, and sailed at a young age on a ship of immigrants from Naples to New York. He fought as a soldier for the United States in the First World War and then settled in New England. During his entire life, he was active, raking leaves and shoveling snow until he died at age 110. Antonio Pierro also said exercise was his secret. He once told a reporter: "If you don't have exercise, you get stiff, you're not worth anything."[3]

There are many such examples. In our family, it was grand-father August. He lived in the country outside Cologne, Germany, and worked as a carpenter at a time when craftsmen took a nap in the hay after lunch. Every day, August took an evening stroll for an hour, and he lived to be 98 years old.

These long and fulfilled lives are more than just chance. Epidemiological studies of thousands of men and women have shown that the regular use of our muscles is the only means capable of prolonging the human life.[4] Being fit reduces mortality by 50 percent. People who burn 1000 kilocalories per week by additional exercise increase their probability of surviving by 20 percent. And if people become physically active but also quit smoking, they will live eight years longer, on average.

After all, we are born to run. We evolved the ability to run long distances—and this, believes the anthropologist Daniel Lieberman at Harvard University, was crucial for our evolution. When it comes to endurance, we are among the best athletes in the animal kingdom. Leopards, for example, might sprint much faster, but over long distances, the big cats will be worn out before long. Actually, most mammals are not capable of running or trotting for longer than 15 minutes. Chimpanzees, with their bowlegs, come off especially badly. In contrast, humans evolved to become true endurance runners. Thanks to our uncovered skin and our sweat glands, we are able to regulate our body temperature even when we move for an extended time in hot weather. And unlike all the other apes, the human body sports a large gluteal muscle, *Musculus gluteus maximus*, which in biomechanical terms enables us to run. Because our potential for endurance running is genetically hardwired into our bodies, we can utilize it even in old age. "Humans are astonishing athletes," Lieberman says. "They can keep running." And yet physicians traditionally thought older people would not have these capabilities. When older runners started attempting marathons, doctors and organizers wondered whether they would need additional care. But these runners did just fine: older athletes can reach the finish line just as comfortably as the younger ones. It is not age that matters but preparation and fitness.[5] Bob Matteson of Bennington, Vermont, began his running career at age 69. By now this ancient gazelle is in his 90s and belongs to the fastest people of his age group.[6]

The course of our lives is often set in middle age. Good strength of grip and normal weight are predictors for an unusually long life. Conversely, the risk of dying because of cancer increases by 29 percent among sedentary women. If a person does not exercise at all, basic strength decreases every year by 1 to 2 percent. At some point, strength falls short of a certain threshold, leaving the muscles unable to fulfill their function—until finally one day a person is too weak to get up from a chair. Comparing this loss of 1 or 2 percent of strength per year with the gain of 30 to 40 percent that can be achieved by training makes it clear that the potential for renewal amounts to 15 to 20 years, which beats any antiaging remedy by far.

Any person who was born healthy can reap the good effects of exercise. Contrary to common belief, this is little affected by an individual's genetic makeup. The impact of the genes on the life expectancy is much smaller than most people would imagine. A survey among thousands of twins revealed that the physically active member of the pair has a significantly lower mortality than the sedentary sibling.[7]

The proverb that one should choose one's parents carefully in order to have a long, healthy life is becoming less true. Genes may determine the way we age by 30 percent;[8] the environment determines the rest. To a large extent, we determine how fast we age. Apart from smoking, it is above all disuse of the body that shortens lives. This weakens the potency of men, makes us vulnerable to stress, steals our healthy sleep, and increases the number of illnesses we get.

WORKING OUT FOR POTENCY

It was the first day of June 1889 when the neurologist Charles Edouard Brown-Sequard declared at the Biological Society of France in Paris that he had discovered a fountain of youth and had already tested it. The result, the 72-year-old professor claimed, was nothing but a sensation. Brown-Sequard said he felt physically strong and mentally awakened. He had gotten rid of his constipation and urinated again like in his young days, in a high arch. The professor was convinced these improvements were due to an extract he had prepared from the testes of guinea pigs and dogs, and subsequently injected into his own body. As it turned out, this supposed antiaging regimen had, if anything, a placebo effect because its recipe was simply too weak to work. Nevertheless, Brown-Sequard had founded a new field dealing with the production and effects of hormones, today known as endocrinology. Furthermore, his hunch that the testes are an important reloading point for hormones was subsequently proven right.[9]

By 1935, chemists were able to simulate the work of the glands by synthesizing testosterone in the laboratory. Normally, it is produced in the male body but also—in smaller amounts—in the female body. It promotes the maturation of the male reproductive organs; helps with the production of new sperm; and, in both sexes, strengthens the libido.

Furthermore, testosterone acts as an anabolic hormone and increases the buildup of proteins in cells, enabling muscle growth, for example. Small wonder that testosterone and the similar hormone DHEA are marketed as antiaging products and consumed by many men. Doctors and public-relations people with ties to pharmaceutical companies even invented a disease, which they have named "male menopause," to generate more sales. Due to an age-related decline of testosterone, men supposedly become sluggish, sexually slack, and grumpy.

But in reality, hormone prescriptions help only the drug manufacturer and the prescribing doctor. A study has just shown that neither testosterone nor DHEA enhance well-being when given as drugs. A two-year study of elderly men (using testosterone plaster and DHEA tablets) and women (taking DHEA tablets alone) tested these products. Although this resulted in higher hormone levels, it did not affect muscle strength, aerobic capacity, or quality of life. There was no trace of an antiaging effect.[10]

Obviously these hormones are helpful and effective only if produced by the body. This natural buildup is stimulated by exercise. This has been shown time and again by researchers like John McKinlay and his colleagues of the New England

Research Institutes in Watertown, Massachusetts. In the 1980s they randomly contacted more than 1,700 men between 40 and 70 years of age. Over time, the researchers assessed the health of those men via questionnaires and by measuring their hormone levels. On the one hand, the researchers found that the level of male sex hormones incrementally decreases over the course of time; the testosterone level goes down by about 1 percent every year. On the other hand, testosterone level is significantly influenced by lifestyle. Heavy smokers and people who drink a lot of alcohol have lower hormone levels. Inactive, obese men also have a level 10 to 15 percent below that of physically active men of the same age.[11]

Men suffering from hot flashes often turned out to be sedentary heavyweights. The impact of obesity and other adverse lifestyle factors is roughly as big as the impact of natural aging.[12] Thus, McKinlay concludes that male menopause is nothing but a myth, the symptoms more likely to be caused by laziness and an unhealthy lifestyle.

So if men want to boost their testosterone, they simply have to become active. Several studies examined what happened when men at age of 70 began to work out. Unsurprisingly, their strength increased. But their levels of testosterone and growth hormone rose, too. Whereas the hormone production of fit men responds especially strongly to stimuli, formerly inactive men profit, too. Sedentary men aged 66 to 76 training just for one hour on a stationary bike have seen their level of testosterone go up by 23 percent.[13]

Physical activity also helps men suffering from impotence. The condition, also called erectile dysfunction, is seldom the only problem of the affected men. An individual with an erectile dysfunction usually has quite a few other health issues, such as coronary heart disease, impaired circulation of the legs, and strokes—all of which are caused by a lack of physical exercise.

So, is a flaccid penis an indicator for lack of exercise?

Many findings point that way. An elevated body weight is connected with potency problems. The link between impotence and lack of exercise appears to be the endothelium of the blood vessels, which, as we have already seen, is impaired by inactivity. When that happens, the penis is not properly supplied with blood any longer.

Common sense as well as scientific data thus tell us that impotent men need workouts rather than Viagra. Whereas the pills are expensive and have side effects, physical exercise is safe and free.

In the Massachusetts Male Aging Study, John McKinlay and his colleagues followed more than 590 men.[14] At the start of the study, they were middle-aged and all potent. Eight years later, only 83 percent of them had satisfactory erections and, apart from alcohol abuse and smoking, obesity and lack of exercise were the main reasons for the problem. By contrast, some previously sedentary men in the study had adopted an active lifestyle. In comparison to inactive participants, their likelihood of impotence was reduced by 70 percent. "Early adoption of healthy lifestyles may be the best approach to reducing the burden of erectile dysfunction on the health and the well-being of older men," the doctors conclude. Their recommendation? A brisk two-mile walk every day keeps erectile dysfunction away.[15]

The physician Katherine Esposito has used this effect to help men from southern Italy.[16] The 110 participants in her study were all impotent and overweight (BMI of 30 to 49).

They were randomly assigned into two groups. The control group received information about improving their diets and exercise, but it was kept rather unspecific. Over the next two years they were visited bimonthly by the researchers, but no specific individualized program was provided. The men of the intervention group, however, were asked to lose 10 percent of their body weight and were given concrete tips, namely that they should not eat more than 1,700 kilocalories per day and should begin an active life with swimming, ball games, and many walks. Every four to eight weeks, these participants were counseled by nutrition experts and physical educators.

Two years later, Esposito compared the two groups. Although there was no difference between the groups with regard to their eating habits, their activity patterns differed profoundly. Among the men only vaguely instructed about physical activity, the amount of exercise went up from 51 to 84 minutes per week. In the other group, however, the increase was from 48 to 195 minutes per week. The program also affected body weight. Whereas the BMI went down from 36.4 to 35.7 in the first group, the men in the training group lost much more fat; the average BMI declined from 36.9 to 31.2.

This lifestyle change was very beneficial for sexual performance. Whereas 5 percent of the men in the control group were able to overcome their impotence, 31 percent of the exercisers were able to do so. This result fits the data from epidemiological studies, which indicate that 79 out of 100 men with erectile dysfunction are overweight or obese.

Many men do actually intuit the potential exercise has for their potency. That was revealed when the Massachusetts Male Aging Study examined the course of erectile dysfunction.

More than 300 men were followed for nine years, and during this time impotence problems worsened among 33 percent of them. But in 35 percent of the cases the condition had disappeared. These latter men had apparently adopted healthier lifestyles, with less overeating and more sports, and thus had reversed their illness.

The study has two important messages. First, natural aging impairs potency to a much lesser degree than thought. Second, men can overcome penile problems without pills. This is probably not only because of the physiological improvements, which lead to a better blood supply to the erectile tissue. It might also be that exercise helps men to deal better with stress. With less psychological pressure, lust and libido certainly profit. In a true win-win situation, frequent sex enhances fitness and activates the production of hormones—which in turn creates even more desire.

STRIKING BACK AT STRESS

The reason why exercise keeps bodies young and fit is not as evident as it might appear. After all, even moderate use of the muscles leads to an elevated consumption of oxygen—and thereby to an adverse side effect called oxidative stress. In the wake of this stress, highly reactive chemicals are produced, called free radicals, which can damage a cell's DNA.

Fortunately, we are able to protect ourselves against these dangers. As soon as the body is put in motion, a special program is switched on that can neutralize the adverse effects of exercise as well as psychological stress. The gerontologist Suresh

Rattan of University Aarhus in Denmark believes that this protection is created by certain proteins (which, for historical reasons, have the confusing name of "heat shock proteins"). They act as a shield against stress and thus enhance well-being. In the bodies of Stone Age people, this program was probably switched on most of the time. All humans living today have the same system hardwired into their bodies, but it is usually switched off because modern people hardly use their muscles.[17]

The problem is, when this stress shield is turned off, people are still subjected to stress, of a kind that might be even worse than the stress our Stone Age forebears usually had to deal with. Back then, stress always meant that there was an immediate threat and life was in danger. Those situations involve a swift bodily response: energy is released, and the muscles are supplied with glucose. The heart starts beating faster, and blood pressure and breathing frequency increase so that the body can consume more oxygen. Functions that are not needed in life-threatening situations are suppressed: the sex drive, digestion, and the immune system. At the same time, the body is flooded with stress hormones. They ensure that we do not feel pain and sharpen our senses. This system stood the test when our forebears were escaping from mammoths and saber-tooth tigers, and it helps us to this day—for example, should we have to flee a burning house or run away from other dangers.

So far, so good. But there is a problem: today, even when it is not a matter of life and death, stress waves keep rolling in, due especially to the acceleration of daily life that does not allow us to take any rest periods. Many employees can be reached day and night because of cellular phones, e-mail, and text messages. American companies in particular assume they can disturb their employees at any time, even vacations. There has never before been more continuous stress than in the technologically connected job world. Absolute silence and peace, on the other hand, can also be bad. Individuals who have no friends and must live in social isolation are often burdened by stress, too.

In past times, stress lasted only a short while: Either the saber-tooth tiger got you, or not. Nowadays, stress persists the whole day. Furthermore, stress and the corresponding response are uncoupled in sedentary people. The released energy is not converted into action but stays inside the body. Rather than actively defending against threats, the author Tara Parker-Pope concludes: "Now you're just a person with unregulated blood sugar, high blood pressure, blood clots, a depressed sex drive and a buckling immune system."[18] Add to that the effects on the brain. An excess of stress hormones (glucocorticoides from the adrenal gland) impairs nerve cells and causes atrophy in certain brain regions.

The many consequences of stress for the physiology can be measured and expressed in a unit called "allostatic load." Poor, badly educated individuals usually suffer more stress than people who are affluent and have had extensive education. Sleep deprivation and physical inactivity are also associated with an above-average allostatic load.

However, nobody is at the mercy of stress. We can take measures either to minimize it or prevent its more dangerous effects. A social network seems to help against it. People who have an intact family life, are on good terms with their relatives, and have friends are found to have comparatively lower levels of stress hormones in the blood and live longer than the average.

If stress cannot be circumvented or evaded, which is unfortunately often the case, physical activity is the best answer to it. Rodents running on treadmills do not develop brain disorders as quickly as sedentary rodents when put under stress. They appear to be protected by a still poorly understood mechanism against the adverse processes stress can trigger in the brain.[19] From the vantage point of evolution, this makes perfect sense: "Assuming that the stress response is a neuroendocrine mechanism that occurs in anticipation of physical action, then physical activity should be the natural means to prevent the consequences of stress."[20]

That way, the muscles can burn off the excess energy and normalize the glucose level. The immune system starts working better again, probably because exercise increases the number of leucocytes. Though the details of this stress response are not fully understood, its benefits for our health become evident in study after study. Going for a stroll every day keeps rhinitis and sniffles away, for example. Cornelia Ulrich of the University of Washington in Seattle and her colleagues have demonstrated this in a study including overweight and inactive women. Those women who picked up the habit of walking reduced the likelihood of catching a cold by half compared to sedentary women. Ulrich concludes these findings "add a new facet to the growing literature on the health benefits of moderate exercise."[21]

Moderate exercise leads also to more relaxed sleep patterns, which further decreases the stress burden. In tests, people allowed only four hours of sleep for several nights appeared to be testy and responded with elevated levels of stress hormones and glucose in their blood. Once these people were allowed extra sleep—10 to 12 hours per night—the stress signs disappeared.

Exercise's stress-fighting effects amplify each other and prevent us from premature aging. Physical activity reduces the allostatic load, which is connected with a prolonged life expectancy.

MORE HEALTHY DAYS

The steady increase of the average life expectancy is a triumph of civilization. At the same time, health-care experts and even citizens themselves are afraid of this trend. They believe the extended life expectancy could just mean that people are going to have long periods of sickness, and thus they talk about something they call "excess age." In this view, frail seniors would populate nursery homes and hospitals, and the younger generation would have to take care of them.

It was the physician James Fries of Stanford University who most notably began questioning this grim scenario. In the 1980s he published an essay in the *New England Journal of Medicine* that opened a completely new—and very comforting—view on the fact that we all grow old. If it was possible to push the onset of age-related diseases back, Fries suggested, and if this gain was larger than the time gained by the increased life expectancy, those extra years would be free of disease and full of healthy and happy days. Thus the period of frailty that often precedes a death would not get longer and would occur later. Fries has proposed the term "compression of morbidity" to describe this potential change.

Stay Healthy Longer

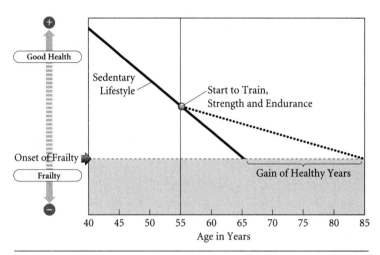

(after Irwin Rosenberg, Biomarkers)

Runners stay in good health longer

The health of runners (members of fitness clubs)
in comparison to sedentary control persons

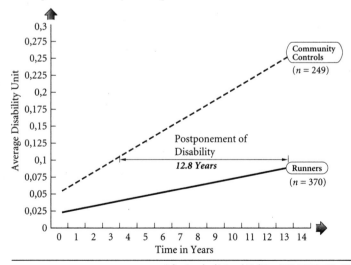

(after Annals of Internal Medicine, 2003, 139, S. 455–459)

When Fries published his ideas, many people dismissed them as wishful thinking. Some even thought it was a downright dangerous view, and that Fries's theory might prevent society from taking measures to deal with an approaching army of sick seniors. By now, many skeptics know better. The compression of morbidity is a valid concept, and we can experience it, if we begin with regular exercise. Fries and his colleagues have shown this in an impressive study[22] that compared 538 people who run regularly (most of them members of a running club) to 423 sedentary people, recruited from the employees at Stanford University. The participants were age 50 or older when the study began. The researchers tracked them for 21 years.

According to their findings, regular running dramatically slows down the effects of aging. Elderly runners, now in their 70s and 80s, have fewer disabilities, a longer span of active life, and were half as likely as non-runners to die early deaths. Nineteen years into the study, 34 percent of non-runners had died compared with 15 percent of runners. At the beginning of the study, the runners ran an average of about four hours a week. After 21 years, their running time declined to an average of 76 minutes a week, but they were still seeing health benefits from running. Both study groups became more disabled after 21 years of aging, but for runners the onset of disability was later. "Runners' initial disability was 16 years later than non-runners,'" Fries says. "By and large, the runners have stayed healthy."[23]

The data refer to avid runners. But what about white-collar workers who stop using their bodies by age 30? Is there something like a point of no return, after which the disuse of the body cannot be made up for?

The uplifting answer given by science is: no. Study after study has revealed that even old and habitually sedentary people still can reap the benefits of exercise if they simply put themselves in motion. These late bloomers complain less often about ailments and need fewer medical treatments. Even individuals at ages 70 to 80, who were almost disabled because of lack of exercise, can overcome ailments by systematic training.

James Fries got it right. In our aging societies, regular exercise can push the onset of diseases back to a later point in life, thus multiplying the number of happy and healthy days. Nobody can avoid growing old. But we can do a lot to keep ourselves from growing old in bad shape.

14

Panacea for Every Day

In THE SOUTHERN PART OF THE CANADIAN PROVINCE OF ONTARIO there is a long-lived group of people whose lives involve heavy physical labor. They belong to a Christian denomination whose founders immigrated to America in the eighteenth century from the Alsace region, the German-speaking parts of Switzerland and Germany. To this day they talk in a German dialect and call themselves "Amische" or "amische Leit." They hold the belief that they are in this world, but not of this world, and live like their ancestors did roughly 200 years ago.

While other Amish people in North America, such as those in Pennsylvania, have incrementally adopted certain technologies, like tractors, the approximately 500 Amish of the Ontario settlement refrain to this day from using any new technologies—which has bestowed an enviable vitality upon them.

This was revealed by David Bassett, of the University of Tennessee in Knoxville, and the anthropologist Gertrude Huntington, of the University of Michigan in Ann Arbor, who studied the level of physical activity in this group. "The people stay active when they are much older than 80," says Huntington.

Usually the Amish from this settlement in Ontario avoid any contact with the surrounding world of the "English." They are happy that their houses and farms, in a sparsely populated area approximately 40 miles south of the vibrant city of Toronto, are overlooked by the rest of the world. Here, no visitors show up to gawk at them, and no one takes photos when they travel the gravel roads in their horse-drawn buggies.

But in this case 48 women and 53 men decided to make an exception. The Amish agreed to physical examinations and carried battery-powered pedometers in their skirts and waistbands for a week.[1] The result: on average, the men took 18,425 steps per day, the women 14,196.

The Amish also kept minutes of their day. Within the weeklong period, the women spent 42 hours on moderate-to-hard physical work and walked for five hours. The men labored for 52 hours and walked for 12 hours. This means that the Amish are six times more active than the average inhabitants of the industrialized world. Just 9 percent of the Amish women, and none of the men, were obese. That makes them much slimmer than their Canadian neighbors (where 15 percent of the population is obese) and the inhabitants of the United States (where 31 percent is obese), despite the fact that, like their German-speaking ancestors, they love to eat substantial meals, with meat, potatoes, gravy, and homemade cakes.

Few would demand to abandon engine power and electricity, which would mean forgoing the use of laundry machines, dishwashers, computers, and cars. And yet we can learn from these Amish people in Ontario. They are so busy with physical activity in their daily life that it wouldn't occur to them to go to a place called a "gym" to do something for their health. The Amish have succeeded in making physical activity a natural part of their daily chores and work. They are puzzled when they find out that there are people around them who die from insufficient use of their bodies.

BUT WHAT ABOUT GENES?

Although many inhabitants of the industrialized world have integrated physical activity and sports into their daily lives and benefit from an even healthier (because less austere) life than the Amish, millions have yet to discover the healing power of exercise. One reason is that many people simply underestimate the potential of their own bodies. If the good physical condition of healthy people is pointed out to ailing people of the same age, many of them will dismiss this comparison as unfair, saying their healthier peers have always been physically active. But this line of thought ignores the fact that the benefits of physical activity can be reaped by every person who was born healthy. The body is more potent than most people can imagine. There is no medical or biological reason to retire at age 62, 65, or 68 because studies have revealed that people who are aware how important physical activity is stay more or less at the same level of health between age 55 and 75.

To the extent that people misjudge the body's capability to rejuvenate, they overrate the influence of their genes on physical constitution. There is no question that, aside from the lifestyle, the genetic makeup affects fitness and physiological reserves. Yet it is revealing how experts view this. The sports physician Aloys Berg of the University Hospital in Freiburg, Germany, concludes that "even if there is an unfavorable predisposition, the individual range is large enough so that lifestyle changes can beneficially influence the emergence of risk factors and the onset of chronic diseases."[2]

Maria Fiatarone Singh, chair of Exercise and Sport Science at the University of Sydney, puts it this way: "However, at least partial escape from a genetic predisposition to type 2 diabetes, stroke, coronary artery disease, hypertension, obesity, and other major scourges of modern civilization is possible with the adoption of realistic doses of physical activity. Much of the typical phenotype of the aged person—a thinning, curved spine, wasted muscles, and bulging abdominal adipose tissue—is more closely related to time spent in a gym than to the passage of years. Furthermore, body composition is still susceptible to change by anabolic stimuli, particularly robust forms of resistance exercise, in the tenth decade of life, despite a lifetime of sedentary behavior."[3] Fiatarone Singh knows what she is talking about. She is the doctor who encouraged people aged 90 and older to do strength training, giving them back their power.

There is no shortage of studies showing the body's potential for renewal. In a study done in Texas in 1966, doctors examined five young men and documented their fitness levels. Thirty years later the procedure was repeated, and it became evident that years of sedentary living had reduced their fitness. Next, the men, now aged 50 to 51, were subjected to 24 weeks of endurance training of moderate intensity with jogging, walking, bicycle riding—with the result that their de-

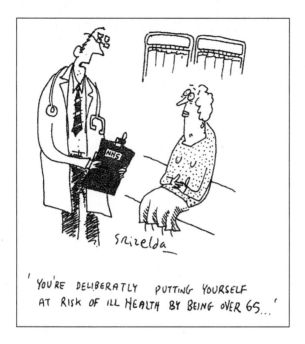

'YOU'RE DELIBERATLY PUTTING YOURSELF AT RISK OF ILL HEALTH BY BEING OVER 65...'

cline was fully reversed, and they reached the same level as 30 years before.

The general public usually ignores this capacity for rejuvenation. Our society denies that older people have physical reserves. This ageism can be seen any time younger people start talking more loudly and using simpler vocabulary when addressing an older person. This discriminating approach can lead to a self-fulfilling prophecy. As a result of being treated like idiots, older people indeed start to walk slower, have impaired hearing, and become prone to cardiovascular diseases.

The psychologist Becca Levy at Yale University in New Haven, Connecticut, has studied this phenomenon among 90 healthy elderly persons. At first she tested the memories of these volunteers, then showed them positive attributes about aging, such as "wise," "alert," "learned," and "sage," and retested them. Afterward, their memories had improved and the participants even walked faster.

To check her findings, Levy showed her subjects such negative words as "decrepit," "senile," "dementia," and "confused," and carried out yet another memory test. Now, their memories were worse, and the participants walked significantly more slowly.[4]

A NEGLECTED REMEDY

Although exercise is one of the most potent and effective remedies in existence, it plays only a small role in medical-school training. For this reason, American doctors rarely recommend exercise. Even though some doctors do prescribe exercise, physicians can make a much greater profit with drugs and operations. Faith in the power of medicine is another reason why people tend to underestimate the value of exercise. The number of back surgeries has increased dramatically in recent years, while pills for high blood pressure and drugs to lower cholesterol have sales in the billions of dollars. This fuels the medical industry and might meet the expectations of many patients, but it still amounts to nothing more than tinkering with the symptoms.

This turn toward big pharmacology and invasive medical procedures is promoted by faulty financial incentives in the health-care system. One example is a booming procedure called angioplasty, which is the mechanical widening of a narrowed or totally obstructed blood vessel. In about 80 percent of these procedures a small tube, a stent, is inserted to keep the vessel open. However, in 20 to 40 percent of angioplasties, the affected area becomes narrowed again.

These results are less good than those produced by a landmark trial published in the journal *Circulation*.[5] In this exercise program the patients had fewer complications, less pain, and their treatment was cheaper. Ignoring these impressive results, many physicians continue to recommend and carry out angioplasties. The procedure, introduced in 1977 by a German radiologist, has grown into an $8 billion annual industry in the United States alone, where it is performed 650,000 to 1 million times a year.[6]

Even when doctors are willing to use the new science of healing through exercise, they often find that patients would prefer an invasive procedure and drug regimen, rather than the supposedly silly advice of bicycling 30 minutes a day. Obese patients and smokers who cannot be coaxed into changing their behavior repeatedly frustrate such doctors.

Many middle-aged people cannot envision the long-term repercussions of complete physical inactivity—a life of continual ailments and increasing weight gain: "Obesity is not like running through a minefield, which kills you all at once or lets you run through it unscathed," says David Allison, a biostatistician at the University of Alabama, Birmingham. "Instead, your risk increases over time. What you die of is the accumulated effects from years of obesity."[7]

Fiatarone Singh emphasizes the absurdity of medical practices in industrialized countries: "Imagine the 85-year-old woman with cachexia [a wasting condition], congestive heart failure, osteoporosis, depression, recurrent falls, type 2 diabetes, hypertension, peripheral vascular disease, osteoarthritis, insomnia, and functional decline. Whereas a pharmaceutical approach to most of these problems is possible, and would be the usual course of action, the potential for iatrogenesis [further problems caused by the medical treatment], burden for the patient, and cost of such treatment is substantial. If exercise were taken seriously by her doctor, however, and used to its full potential, all of her clinical problems could be addressed in part by the prescription of a tailored exercise regime, which could reduce to a minimum the number and doses of medications needed."[8]

The uses of exercise to treat diseases are so novel that many physicians are not taking advantage of them. Yet the paradigm is shifting, and many signs indicate that a new mind-set is gaining ground. In Seattle, the YMCA and Fred Hutchinson Cancer Research Center now offer an exercise program for cancer survivors. The 10-week program, called Exercise and Thrive, is available free to adults who have completed cancer treatment, regardless of where they were treated.[9]

The American College of Sports Medicine and the American Medical Association have now joined forces to launch a program called "Exercise Is Medicine," designed to encourage patients to incorporate physical activity and exercise into their daily routines and to urge doctors to prescribe exercise to their patients.[10] "Why physicians are so quick to accept research data on expensive medications while essentially ignoring even stronger data on the benefits of physical activity is at the core of this program," says Robert Sallis, a past president of the American College of Sports Medicine. "We already advise against smoking; recommending exercise should be no different."[11]

In Great Britain, general practitioners are turning to exercise therapy to help people with depression. The Mental Health Foundation, based in London and Glasgow, says that 22 percent of doctors now prescribe exercise therapy as one of their most common treatments for depression, compared to only 5 percent three years ago.[12]

Having a family doctor talk to patients about the importance of exercise appears to be the most effective way to get people going. It just takes some unorthodox but simple steps. What if doctors gathered their sedentary patients on a certain afternoon of the week and took them on a walk? Patients would be astounded how much their glucose level drops after just a few minutes of brisk walking.

In hospitals and nursing homes, the time is also ripe for change. Being bedridden should no longer be regarded as an inevitable fate but as a side effect of bed rest. Mobilizing patients at risk of being bedridden could be achieved with more and better-educated nursing personnel and improved facilities, including better-designed furniture and rooms. In hospitals especially, there should be more time and money available for training to reverse the disastrous consequences of too much bed rest.

LESS IS MORE

When people decide to change their lives, they often set themselves unrealistic goals they cannot achieve. They want to become athletic and slim in no time. They go out and buy

Energy Expenditure per Hour

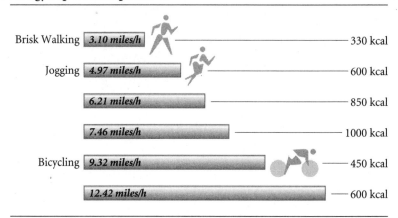

Brisk Walking	3.10 miles/h	330 kcal
Jogging	4.97 miles/h	600 kcal
	6.21 miles/h	850 kcal
	7.46 miles/h	1000 kcal
Bicycling	9.32 miles/h	450 kcal
	12.42 miles/h	600 kcal

(after Marc Ziegler et al. MMW-Fortschr. Med. 2004; 8)

sneakers and sporting clothes, sign up at the gym, and start with great enthusiasm. This period of euphoria usually lasts four weeks. Then exercise turns into a burden. Month after month, gym fees are charged to credit cards whose owners hardly work out anymore.

There is no need to have such ambitious targets. Fortunately, science shows that surprisingly small amounts of exercise suffice to put health and well-being on the right track. Formerly, exercise recommendations were based on the assumption that sweat-inducing drudgery was needed to achieve therapeutic effects. But a recent review of 44 studies revealed that most of the good effects start appearing at an intensity corresponding to the burning of 1000 kilocalories per week. Among sedentary adults, even the expenditure of just 500 to 800 kilocalories produces slight improvements.[13]

One general recommendation is to perform 30 minutes of moderate activity, five or more days per week;[14] the exercise can be brisk walking, jogging, or bicycle riding. This amount is apparently enough to meet the evolutionary needs hardwired into our bodies, which are still adapted to the Stone Age. If a person walks for 30 minutes, he or she burns 200 to 250 kilocalories. Doing this five times a week, plus some work in the garden and home, and a person uses nearly 2000 kilocalories per week.

This surprisingly low minimal requirement has two advantages. First, the risk of injury is extremely low, and one need not fear sore muscles. The benefit of this low-intensity exercise is much greater than the potential harm. One can start slowly and increase intensity step by step. People who were completely inactive for years, or who are already sick or ailing in some way, can reclaim their bodies through exercise, though they should talk to a physician before starting to set up an individual training program.

Second, one can get small bits of exercise that in turn add up to the recommended daily total. Each errand we run and each chore we do helps. Weeding, vacuuming, sweeping the sidewalk, climbing stairs, walking to the grocery store: if we integrate such activities into our daily lives, we can reach calorie expenditures large enough to improve existing medical conditions and stave off further diseases.

It is fascinating to see that these good effects often multiply and improve other aspects of life. After adopting an active lifestyle, many people abandon other bad habits; they switch to a balanced diet, reduce the number of cigarettes they smoke, or quit smoking altogether. Furthermore, they sleep better and—because they lead by example—increase the activity of their children.

FIT IS MORE IMPORTANT THAN FAT

Finally, we benefit from exercise even when we are not losing weight. Overweight men are especially protected against heart attacks by physical activity. Similarly, women who are overweight but active have a slightly lower risk for heart disease than slim but inactive women. Being overweight does not harm one's health—as long as a heavy body is kept in motion.

This is also the message of a recent study by doctors and physiologists at the University of South Carolina in Columbia.[15] They measured the body mass index, waist circumference, and body fat of more than 2,600 adults aged 60 years or older, assessed their fitness by a treadmill exercise test, and followed the group for 12 years. "Fitness was a significant mortality predictor in older adults, independent of overall or abdominal adiposity," the scientists reported in the *Journal of the American Medical Association*. Active heavyweights live longer than inactive slim people—fit is more important than fat. And nobody needs to become an athlete. According to the study, walking for 30 minutes on most days of the week already increases the chances to "achieve a healthy lifestyle and to enjoy longer life in better health."

To be sure, these effects can be enhanced. Exercise and health are directly correlated; the more we use our muscles, the bigger the gain. Imagine 60 minutes of moderate exercise, five or more days per week—what a treat for body and soul that would that be! This program would also be the right one to fully prevent colon and breast cancer, ideally combined with light strength training two or more days per week.

Still, one should not overtrain the body because there can be too much of a good thing. Regular exercise corresponding to an expenditure of 3,500 kilocalories per week or more can lead to adverse effects.[16]

Those trying to lose weight by starving themselves for long periods are bound to fail. Our Stone Age genes are programmed in such a way that we long for the juiciest ham and the sweetest fruit. Dieting fads have come and gone for the past 50 years, but a miracle regimen has yet to be found. If a person manages to be on a diet for 15 weeks, he or she can lose up to 24 pounds. Yet the effect usually vanishes within three to five years. It would be much smarter to exercise more while keeping food intake the same or reducing it slightly. If we burn 700 kilocalories more than we consume every day, our weight inevitably goes down, by about one pound per week. I would recommend documenting this by recording one's weight every morning.

A WAY OF LIFE

Physical exercise can help us, whatever we do and wherever we go, as long as we allow it to become our permanent companion. The magic formula is to do a little every day and to establish well-being in small but constant steps. At stake is the maintenance of our bodies. If we asked our dentist which teeth we should floss, he would answer: only those you want to keep. The same is true for physical activity: move those muscles you want to keep.

There are easy ways to make family life more mobile. To start with, children should not have their own television sets in their rooms, and the one in the living room should be switched off most of the time. In our house in Arlington, Massachusetts, there are three children and no television. Having been brought up in Europe, I am puzzled to see that many American households have one television set in most of the rooms and, even more disturbing, that the television is sometimes used to babysit toddlers. Americans spend nine times as many leisure hours in front of a screen than being physically active. As we saw earlier, the more time people spend in front of a screen, the more likely they are to develop type 2 diabetes.[17]

The pediatrician Thomas Robinson at Stanford University examined 192 children at two elementary schools. The students at one of the schools were restricted at home to a maximum of one hour per day watching television. The students of the other had no limit—and seven months later they were more than two pounds heavier and their waistlines had increased by an average of one inch.[18]

Another way to get started is to begin with small changes, like 60 seconds of exercise per day. This might seem ridiculous, but the trick is to train two minutes per day in the second week, three minutes per day in the third week, and so on. Half a year later, you will be a presentable athlete and need only to maintain your level. There are also many ways to integrate muscle use with daily life: walk your children to school; avoid escalators and elevators; switch to public transportation and get off the train or bus a few stops earlier, walking the remaining distance. People living in Manhattan are slimmer than the average American, no doubt in part because they walk more. Also, get rid of your second (and third) car and see if you can commute to work by bike. Or join community groups that engage in walking and other physical activities.

When it comes to judging the amount of exercise we get, it's human nature that we tend to deceive ourselves. We perceive even decades of inactivity as an atypical period that will soon be over: "Once I get a promotion . . . once the baby is older . . . once we move nearer to the city." We persistently think of ourselves as more athletic than we actually are. Perhaps we should follow the example of the Amish who agreed to walk around with pedometers. The devices cost around $15 to $20, sense body motion, and count footsteps. This count is converted into distance by knowing the length of your normal stride. Wearing a pedometer and recording your daily steps and distance can be a good motivating tool. If you have taken about 10,000 steps by evening, you can put your feet up and be happy—you have done your daily stint.

THE GLOBAL CHALLENGE

Physical inactivity is estimated to cause 2 million deaths worldwide annually, according to the World Health Organization. At least 60 percent of the global population fails to achieve its minimum recommendation of 30 minutes of moderate-intensity physical activity daily, and 17 percent are completely inactive.[19] Meanwhile, health-care costs in the United States and many other industrialized countries are escalating. Nations with universal health care have to pay more for coverage. In those without such coverage, as in the United States, millions of Americans cannot afford insurance, and there is no end of this cost explosion in sight. Dealing with the consequences of physical inactivity is a major part of health costs. In the United States, about $400 billion is spent each year to treat heart disease alone. At the same time, epidemiological studies show that at least one-third of all heart attacks would be avoided if people walked briskly 2.5 hours per week.

As for metabolic disorders, the consequences of not moving are even worse: 91 percent of all cases of type 2 diabetes can be traced back to lifestyle issues. People smoke, they overeat—and they let their muscles waste away. If we could magically remove the problem of physical inactivity from the world, the financial crisis we see in our health-care systems would be far easier to resolve.

So, should people asking for health insurance continue to have the right to be sedentary? In the wake of the emerging science of motion, doctors have started posing such questions: "From childhood, when unhealthy food habits begin and sedentary lifestyles are copied from parents, people must be educated about the risks of inactivity and overeating. The degree to which unhealthy behavior is regarded as a private issue should be publicly discussed," state the cardiologists Rainer Hambrecht and Stefan Gielen in an essay in the medical journal *The Lancet*. "A balance needs to be struck between a reasonable minimum effort on the part of the individual to reduce the health-care costs associated with their lifestyle, and intrusion of an investigative health-care system into personal lifestyle."[20]

In this vein, one option would be to make physically inactive people pay for their own medication if they are unwilling to change their lifestyles. One example would be high blood pressure, which is a direct consequence of inactivity and can be reversed through exercise. If a patient opts not to use this proven and cheap remedy and prefers to take drugs, why, then, should he not pay for them out of his own pocket?

The precondition for such an approach would be that patients be given professional consultations about the benefits of exercise. Because physical activity has turned out to be one of the most broadly effective therapies known, one without the adverse side effects of some drugs, it is absurd that there are still no real incentives to make doctors prescribe this miracle remedy.

Of course, it would be naive to assume that people will start exercising solely because they want to help our troubled health-care system. Regulations asserting that exercise is something like a duty of each citizen are unrealistic and undesirable in a free society. But becoming informed about the emerging role of exercise as preventive and curative medicine should be our duty to each other. Each of us can walk along this path. It's never too late, and every step will be rewarded.

NOTES

CHAPTER 1: THE HEALING POWER OF EXERCISE

1. Personal communication; I visited Wayne Sandler in his practice in Los Angeles in the summer of 2005.

2. Personal communication and talk by Carolyn Kaelin in Wellesley, Massachusetts, fall 2005; see also Carolyn Kaelin with Francesca Coltrera, *Living Through Breast Cancer* (New York: McGraw-Hill, 2005).

3. Wildor Hollmann and others, "Körperliche Aktivität und Gesundheit," *Blickpunkt Der Mann* 3 (2006): 11–15.

4. Christoph Schmidt-Hieber, Peter Jonas, and Josef Bischofberger, "Enhanced Synaptic Plasticity in Newly Generated Granule Cells of the Adult Hippocampus," *Nature* 429 (2004): 184–187.

5. Personal communication. See also the review paper by Henriette van Praag, "Neurogenesis and Exercise: Past and Future Directions," *Neuromolecular Medicine* 10 (2008): 128–140.

6. Jean Marx, "Preventing Alzheimer's: A Lifelong Commitment?" *Science* 309 (2005): 864–866.

7. Michael Babyak and others, "Exercise Treatment for Major Depression: Maintenance of Therapeutic Benefit at 10 Months," *Psychosomatic Medicine* 62 (2000): 633–638.

8. Nicola T. Lautenschlager and others, "Effect of Physical Activity on Cognitive Function in Older Adults at Risk for Alzheimer

Disease," *Journal of the American Medical Association* 300 (2008): 1027–1037.

9. B. K. Pedersen and B. Saltin, "Evidence for Prescribing Exercise as Therapy in Chronic Disease," *Scandinavian Journal of Medicine & Science in Sports* 16 (Suppl.1, 2006): 3–63.

10. Carol Derby and others, "Modifiable Risk Factors and Erectile Dysfunction: Can Lifestyle Changes Modify Risk?" *Urology* 56 (2000): 302–306.

11. Personal communication, June 6, 2008.

12. Thorsten Schulz, Christiane Peters, and Horst Michna, "Bewegungstherapie und Sport in der Krebstherapie und-nachsorge," *Deutsche Zeitschrift für Onkologie* 37, no. 4 (2005): 159–168.

13. The life-prolonging effect was just confirmed by two new studies among women with breast cancer: Crystal N. Holick, et al., "Physical Activity and Survival After Diagnosis of Invasive Breast Cancer," *Cancer Epidemiology Biomarkers & Prevention* 17 (2008): 379–386; and Melinda Irwin, et al., "Influence of Pre-and Postdiagnosis Physical Activity on Mortality in Breast Cancer Survivors: The Health, Eating, Activity and Lifestyle Study," *Journal of Clinical Oncology* 26 (2008): 3958–3964.

14. Personal communication, July 1, 2008.

15. Rainer Hambrecht, "Sport als Therapie," (Physical Exercise as Treatment Strategy) *Herz* 29 (2004): 381–390.

16. Amy A. Hakim and others, "Effects of Walking on Mortality Among Nonsmoking Retired Men," *New England Journal of Medicine* 338 (1998): 94–99.

17. Heinz Mechling, "Körperlich-sportliche Aktivität und erfolgreiches Altern," *Bundesgesundheitsbl–Gesundheitsforsch–Gesundheitsschutz* 48 (2005): 899–905.

18. Randolph Nesse and George Williams, *Why We Get Sick* (New York: Vintage Books, 1995).

19. Lynn Cherkas and others, "The Association Between Physical Activity in Leisure Time and Leukocyte Telomere Length," *Archives of Internal Medicine* 168 (2008): 154–158.

20. Frank Booth and others, "Waging War on Physical Inactivity: Using Modern Molecular Ammunition Against an Ancient Enemy," *Journal of Applied Physiology* 93 (2002): 3–30.

21. Heinz Mechling, "Körperlich-sportliche Aktivität und erfolgreiches Altern," *Bundesgesundheitsbl–Gesundheitsforsch–Gesundheitsschutz* 48 (2005): 899–905.

22. The physician Barron H. Lerner published an essay on the role of coincidence in medicine: *New York Times*, September 19, 2006.

23. Allen Warburton and others, "Health Benefits of Physical Activity: The Evidence," *Canadian Medical Association Journal* 174, no.6 (2006): 801–809.

24. Annette Becker, "Activating Medicine—A New Approach to Illness" (Schonungslose Medizin–Der neue Umgang mit dem Kranksein), *Zeitschrift für Allgemeinmedizin* 82 (2006): 338–342.

25. Rüdiger Reer, et al., "Bewegungstherapie als therapeutisches Prinzip," *Bundesgesundheitsbl–Gesundheitsforsch Gesundheitsschutz* 48 (2005): 841–847.

26. Ibid.

27. Linn Goldberg and Diane Elliot, *The Healing Power of Exercise* (New York: John Wiley, 2000).

28. Thomas S. Kuhn, *The Structure of Scientific Revolutions*, 3rd ed. (Chicago: University of Chicago Press, 1996).

29. Reer and others.

CHAPTER 2: THE DANGERS OF GOING TO BED

1. Annette Becker, "Activating Medicine—A New Approach to Illness" (Schonungslose Medizin—Der neue Umgang mit dem Kranksein), *Zeitschrift für Allgemeinmedizin* 82 (2006): 338–342.

2. It was Sir Richard Asher's intention "to justify placing beds and graves in the same category." He concluded his report about the "dangers of going to bed" with the following poem:
"Teach us to live that we may dread
Unnecessary time in bed.

Get people up and we may save
Our patients from an early grave."
Richard Asher, "The Dangers of Going to Bed," *British Medical Journal* 2 (1947): 967–968.

3. Thomas Mann, *The Magic Mountain,* trans. H. T. Lowe-Porter (New York: The Modern Library, 1992).

4. Jules Romains, *Knock,* trans. James B. Gidney (New York: Barron's Educational Series, 1962).

5. Chris Allen and others, "Bed Rest: A Potentially Harmful Treatment Needing More Careful Evaluation," *The Lancet* 354 (1999): 1229–1233.

6. Ibid.

7. Thomas Gill and others, "Hospitalization, Restricted Activity, and the Development of Disability Among Older Persons," *Journal of the American Medical Association* 292 (2004): 2115–2124.

8. Angelika Abt-Zegelin, "Prävention von Bettlägerigkeit," *Die Schwester Der Pfleger* 3 (2006): 210–213.

9. Almut Schmid and others, "Nährstoff-und Bewegungsmangel im Altenheim weitverbreitet," *Geriatrie Journal* 1–2 (2001): 31–34.

10. Abt-Zegelin, 210–213.

11. Almut Schmid and others, 31–34.

12. Paul Corcoran, "Use It or Lose It—The Hazards of Bed Rest and Inactivity," *Rehabilitation Medicine—Adding Life to Years*, Special Issue of *The Western Journal of Medicine* 154 (1991): 536–538.

13. B. Saltin, G. Blomqvist, J. H. Mitchell, and others, "Response to Exercise After Bed Rest and After Training: A Longitudinal Study of Adaptive Changes in Oxygen Transport and Body Composition," *Circulation* 37/38, suppl. VII (1968): VII-1–VII-78.

14. B. K. Pedersen and B. Saltin, "Evidence for Prescribing Exercise as Therapy in Chronic Disease," *Scandinavian Journal of Medicine & Science in Sports* 16, suppl. 1 (2006): 3–63.

15. Saltin, Blomqvist, Mitchell, and others, VII-1–VII-78.

16. Walter Bortz, "The Disuse Syndrome," *The Western Journal of Medicine* 141 (1984): 691–694.

17. Angelika Zegelin, "Festgenagelt Sein—Der Prozess des Bettlägerig-werdens durch allmähliche Ortsfixierung," *Pflege* 18 (2005): 281–288.

18. Corcoran, 536–538.

19. Becker, 338–342.

20. Irwin Rosenberg granted me an interview in October 2005 when he actually read to me from his 1991 book, saying that its message is still valid and timely. See also William Evans and Irwin Rosenberg with Jacqueline Thompson, *Biomarkers—The 10 Keys to Prolonging Vitality* (New York: Fireside Books, 1991).

CHAPTER 3: UNEMPLOYED BODIES, NEW DISEASES

1. Hans Kraus and Wilhelm Raab, *Hypokinetic Disease—Disease Produced by Lack of Exercise* (Springfield, Illinois: Charles C. Thomas, 1961).

2. H. Mellerowicz, "Bewegungsmangel–und seine Folgen," *Zeitschrift für Öffentliches Gesundheitwesen* 29.11 (1967): 512–519.

3. Ibid.

4. The figures refer to the year 2000. www.who.int/dietphysicalactivity/publications/facts/pa/en/.

5. William Haskell, "Sport, Bewegung und Gesundheit," *Der Orthopäde* 29 (2000): 930–935.

6. American Academy of Pediatrics, "Children, Adolescents, and Television," *Pediatrics* 107 (2001): 423–426.

7. Haskell, 930–935.

8. Frank Booth and Darrell Neufer, "Exercise Controls Gene Expression," *American Scientist* (January 2005).

9. http://www.cdc.gov/nccdphp/dnpa/bmi/index.htm; to calculate the BMI you divide your weight (in kilograms) by the square of your height (in meters). Alternatively you can divide your weight (in pounds) by the square of your height (in inches), then multiply with the factor 703.

10. Paul was one of the patients in the rehabilitation facility Insula for obese adolescents in Berchtesgaden, Bavaria. *Der Spiegel* 51 (2000).

11. Peter Gluckman and Mark Hanson, *Mismatch—Why Our World No Longer Fits Our Bodies* (Oxford: Oxford University Press, 2006).

12. *The Boston Globe*, December 26, 2006.

13. S. Boyd Eaton and Stanley Eaton, "An Evolutionary Perspective on Human Physical Activity: Implications for Health," *Comparative Biochemistry and Physiology. Part A, Molecular & Integrative Physiology* 136.1 (2003): 153–159.

CHAPTER 4: WALKING OFF DIABETES

1. Diabetes in Indigenous People Forum in Melbourne convened on November 12, 2006.

2. *Spiegel Online*, November 13, 2006.

3. Manu Chakravarthy and Frank Booth, "Eating, Exercise, and 'thrifty' Genotypes: Connecting the Dots Toward an Evolutionary Understanding of Modern Chronic Diseases," *Journal of Applied Physiology* 96 (2004): 3–10.

4. S. Jay Olshansky and others, "A Potential Decline in Life Expectancy in the United States in the 21st Century," *New England Journal of Medicine* 352 (2007): 1138–1145.

5. Derrick Jackson, "Diabetes—The Silent Killer Among Us," *The Boston Globe*, September 30, 2006.

6. Thea Shavlakadze and Miranda Grounds, "Of Bears, Frogs, Meat, Mice, and Men: Complexity of Factors Affecting Skeletal Muscle Mass and Fat," *BioEssays* 28 (2006): 994–1009.

7. Sally Squires, "Fat Cats, Poor Prognosis," *The Washington Post*, September 12, 2006.

8. Frank Booth and Darrell Neufer, "Exercise Controls Gene Expression," *American Scientist* (January 2005).

9. Not only in the United States and in Germany, but all over the world type 2 diabetes is rapidly spreading. In 1985 it is estimated there were 30 million patients worldwide. Now, the number appears to be 230 million, and for 2026 a number of 350 million is expected (unless action is taken). These figures surfaced at the 42nd annual meeting of

the European Association for the Study of Diabetes in Copenhagen, Denmark.

10. www.nih.gov/about/researchresultsforthepublic/Type2Diabetes .pdf.

11. Christian Roberts and James Barnard, "Effects of Exercise and Diet on Chronic Disease," *Journal of Applied Physiology* 98 (2005): 3–30.

12. Press release from the National Institute of Diabetes and Digestive and Kidney Diseases, February 6, 2002, www.nih.gov/news/pr/feb2002/hhs-06.htm.

13. Javier Ibañez and others, "Twice-Weekly Progressive Resistance Training Decreases Abdominal Fat and Improves Insulin Sensitivity in Older Men With Type 2 Diabetes," *Diabetes Care* 28 (2005): 662–667.

14. Clare Gillies and others, "Pharmacological and Lifestyle Interventions to Prevent or Delay Type 2 Diabetes in People with Impaired Glucose Tolerance: Systematic Review and Meta-Analysis," *British Medical Journal,* doi:10.1136/bmj.39063.689375.55 (published January 19, 2007).

15. Frank Hu and others, "Elevated Risk of Cardiovascular Disease Prior to Clinical Diagnosis of Type 2 Diabetes," *Diabetes Care* 25 (2002): 1129–1134.

CHAPTER 5: MUSCLES AND METABOLISM

1. William Evans and Irwin Rosenberg with Jacqueline Thompson, *Biomarkers—The 10 Keys to Prolonging Vitality* (New York: Fireside Books, 1991).

2. Ibid.

3. Ibid.

4. Aloys Berg and others, "Mehr Bewegung für alle–Ansätze zur Veränderung von Lebensstil und Gesundheitsprofil," *Kinder-und Jugendmedizin* 4 (2004): 139–145.

5. Markus Schülke and others, "Myostatin Mutation Associated with Gross Muscle Hypertrophy in a Child," *New England Journal of Medicine* 350 (2004): 2682–2688.

6. Henriette Pilegaard and others, "Transcriptional Regulation of Gene Expression in Human Skeletal Muscle During Recovery from Exercise," *American Journal of Physiology, Endocrinology and Metabolism* 279, issue 4 (2000): E806-E814.

7. Jouko Karjalainen and others, "Muscle Fiber-Type Distribution Predicts Weight Gain and Unfavorable Left Ventricular Geometry: A 19-Year Follow-Up Study," *BMC Cardiovascular Disorders* 6 (2006): 2.

8. Personal communication. I interviewed Dr. Williams in September 2006 in Boston when he gave a talk at Harvard Medical School.

9. Evans and Rosenberg with Thompson.

10. Aloys Berg and others, "Gewichtskontrolle ist nicht nur FdH," *MMW—Fortschritte der Medizin* 27–28 (2004): 636–639.

11. John Todd and R. J. Robinson, "Osteoporosis and Exercise," *Postgrad Medical Journal* 79 (2003): 320–323.

12. Evans and Rosenberg with Thompson.

13. The definition of what is a cholesterol value too high should be met with skepticism because it was drafted by doctors with ties to the pharmaceutical industry. The threshold value for cholesterol was many times lowered in the Western countries, so that the majority of Americans and Europeans now have cholesterol values that are supposedly too high, including normal-weight people who exercise. See Jörg Blech, *Pushing Pills and Inventing Disease* (London: Routledge, 2006).

14. William Kraus and others, "Effects of the Amount and Intensity of Exercise on Plasma Lipoproteins," *New England Journal of Medicine* 347 (2002): 1438–1492.

15. Hans-Georg Predel, "Werden Sie Lebensstil-Manager!" *MMW—Fortschritte der Medizin* 47 (2006): 29.

16. Evans and Rosenberg with Thompson.

CHAPTER 6: WHAT THE HEART DESIRES

1. Hans-Georg Predel and Walter Tokarski, "Einfluss Körperlicher Aktivität auf die Menschliche Gesundheit," *Bundesgesundheitsblatt—Gesundheitsforschung—Gesundheitsschutz* 48.8 (2005): 833–840.

2. Rainer Hambrecht, "Sport als Therapie (Physical Exercise as Treatment Strategy)," *Herz*, 29 (2004): 381–390.

3. www.dgpr.de.

4. B. K. Pedersen and B. Saltin, "Evidence for Prescribing Exercise as Therapy in Chronic Disease," *Scandinavian Journal of Medicine & Science in Sports* 16, suppl. 1 (2006): 3–63.

5. A. W. Gardner and E. T. Poehlman, "Exercise Rehabilitation Programs for the Treatment of Claudication Pain: A Meta-Analysis," *Journal of the American Medical Association* 274 (1995): 975–980.

6. Pedersen and Saltin, 3–63.

7. Rainer Hambrecht and others, "Effect of Exercise on Coronary Endothelial Function in Patients with Coronary Artery Disease," *New England Journal of Medicine* 17 (2000): 342, 454–460.

8. Marianne Pynn and others, "Exercise Training Reduces Neointimal Growth and Stabilizes Vascular Lesions after Injury in Apolipoprotein E-Deficient Mice," *Circulation* 109 (2004): 386–392.

9. Romualdo Belardinelli and others, "Effects of Moderate Exercise Training on Thalium Uptake and Contractile Response to Low-Dose Dobutamine of Dysfunctional Myocardium in Patients with Ischemic Cardiomyopathy," *Circulation* 97 (1998): 553–561.

10. Volker Adams and others, "Increase of Circulating Endothelial Progenitor Cells in Patients with Coronary Artery Disease After Exercise-Induced Ischemia," *Arteriosclerosis, Thrombosis, and Vascular Biology* 24 (2004): 684–690.

11. Marcus Sandri and others, "Effects of Exercise and Ischemia on Mobilization and Functional Activation of Blood-Derived Progenitor Cells in Patients with Ischemic Syndromes: Results of 3 Randomized Studies," *Circulation* 111 (2005): 3391–3399. Published online before print June 13, 2005, doi:10.1161/CIRCULATIONAHA.104.527135

12. Personal communication, Rainer Hambrecht. He was at the university hospital in Leipzig and took up a new position in Bremen in June 2006.

13. Sandri and others, 3391–3399.

14. Rainer Hambrecht and others, "Percutaneous Coronary Angioplasty Compared with Exercise Training in Patients with Stable Coronary Artery Disease: A Randomized Trial," *Circulation* 109 (2004): 1371–1378.

15. The costs refer to the improvement by one so-called CCS unit (CCS is for Canadian Cardiovascular Society).

16. Rainer Hambrecht, "Vom Sessel auf das Laufband!" *MMW—Fortschritte der Medizin* 35–36 (2005): 735/26–738/29.

17. *MMW—Fortschritte der Medizin* 48 (2006): 16.

18. The enzymes are superoxide dismutase, catalase, and glutathione peroxidase. See Axel Linke and others, "Antioxidative Effects of Exercise Training in Patients with Chronic Heart Failure," *Circulation* 111 (2005): 1763–1770.

19. Paul Thompson, "Exercise Prescription and Proscription for Patients with Coronary Artery Disease," *Circulation* 112 (2005): 2354–2363.

CHAPTER 7: GROWING BONES

1. Miriam Nelson and others, *Strong Women and Men Beat Arthritis* (New York: Perigee, 2002).

2. Kristin Baker and others, "The Efficacy of Home Based Progressive Strength Training in Older Adults with Knee Osteoarthritis: A Randomized Controlled Trial," *The Journal of Rheumatology* 28 (2001): 1655–1665.

3. Nelson and others.

4. K. S. Thomas and others, "Home Based Exercise Programme for Knee Pain and Knee Osteoarthritis: Randomised Controlled Trial," *British Medical Journal* 325 (2002): 752.

5. B. W. Penninx and others, "Physical Exercise and the Prevention of Disability in Activities of Daily Living in Older Persons with Osteoarthritis," *Archives of Internal Medicine* 161 (2001): 2309–2316.

6. Jean-Michel Brismée and others, "Group and Home-Based Tai Chi in Elderly Subjects with Knee Osteoarthritis: A Randomized Controlled Trial," *Clinical Rehabilitation* 21 (2007): 99–111.

7. Alexandra Kirkley and others, "A Randomized Trial of Arthroscopic Surgery for Osteoarthritis of the Knee," *The New England Journal of Medicine* 359 (2008): 1097–1107.

8. www.mayoclinic.org, accessed June 7, 2008.

9. Klaus-Michael Braumann, *Die Heilkraft der Bewegung* (Munich: Irisiana, 2006).

10. Lars Konradsen and others, "Long Distance Running and Osteoarthrosis," *The American Journal of Sports Medicine* 18 (1990): 379–381.

11. N. E. Lane and others, "The Risk of Osteoarthritis with Running and Aging: A 5-year Longitudinal Study," *Journal of Rheumatology* 20.3 (1993): 461–468.

12. Beat Knechtle and others, "Führt Laufen zu Arthrose?" *Praxis* 95 (2005): 1305–1316.

13. Stefan Gödde, "Rheumatoide Arthritis: Kondition und Sport," *Deutsche Zeitschrift für Sportmedizin* 5 (2004): 137–138.

14. B. K. Pedersen and B. Saltin, "Evidence for Prescribing Exercise as Therapy in Chronic Disease," *Scandinavian Journal of Medicine & Science in Sports* 16, suppl.1 (2006): 3–63.

15. Kevin McCully and others, "Reduced Oxidative Muscle Metabolism in Chronic Fatigue Syndrome," *Muscle Nerve* 19 (1996): 621–625.

16. Kathy Fulcher and Peter White, "Randomised Controlled Trial of Graded Exercise in Patients with the Chronic Fatigue Syndrome," *British Medical Journal* 314 (1997): 1647–1652.

17. Monika Siegrist and others, "Kraftraining an Konventionellen bzw. Oszillierenden Geräten und Wirbelsäulengymnastik in der Prävention der Osteoporose bei Postmenopausalen Frauen," *Deutsche Zeitschrift für Sportmedizin* 7/8 (2006): 182–188.

18. The number relates to women with a femoral neck T score of 2.5 or less; C. Green and others, *Bone Mineral Density Testing: Does the Evidence Support Its Selective Use in Well Women?* (Vancouver, BC: British Columbia Office of Health Technology Assessment, 1997).

19. Steven R. Cummings and others, "Effect of Alendronate on Risk of Fracture in Women with Low Bone Density but Without Vertebral

Fractures: Results from the Fracture Intervention Trial," *Journal of the American Medical Association* 280 (1998): 2077–2082.

20. John Abramson, *Overdosed America* (New York: HarperCollins, 2004).

21. Ibid.

22. Henry Bone and others, "Ten Years' Experience with Alendronate for Osteoporosis in Postmenopausal Women," *New England Journal of Medicine* 350 (2004): 1189–1199.

23. Eckhard Schönau and Oliver Fricke, "Muskel und Knochen—eine funktionelle Einheit," *Deutsches Ärzteblatt* 50 (2006): A3414–A3419.

24. Diane Feskanich and others, "Walking and Leisure-Time Activity and Risk of Hip Fracture in Postmenopausal Women," *Journal of the American Medical Association* 288 (2002): 2300–2306.

25. Press release, University of Freiburg, Germany, March 9, 2004.

26. Ibid.

27. Edward Gregg and others, "Physical Activity and Osteoporotic Fracture Risk in Older Women," *Annals of Internal Medicine* 129 (1998): 81–88.

28. *Der Tagesspiegel*, October 31, 2006.

CHAPTER 8: A SPORTING CURE FOR BACK PAIN

1. I learned about Dr Weinstein's twisted back from a newspaper article and interviewed him subsequently by phone. See also Gina Kolata, "When It's O.K. to Run Hurt," *New York Times*, January 11, 2007.

2. James Weinstein, "Absent from Work: Nature Versus Nurture," *Annals of Internal Medicine* 140 (2004): 142–143.

3. Gordon Waddell and others, "Systematic Reviews of Bed Rest and Advice to Stay Active for Acute Low Back Pain," *British Journal of General Practice* 47 (1997): 647–652.

4. Annette Becker, "Schonungslose Medizin—Der neue Umgang mit dem Kranksein," *Zeitschrift für Allgemeinmedizin* 82 (2006): 338–342.

5. Jan Hildebrandt and S. Mense, "Rückenschmerzen–ein ungelöstes Problem," *Der Schmerz* 6 (2001): 411–412.

6. Steffen Heger, "Zur Psychosomatik des Failed-Back-Syndroms: Warum Rückenschmerzen chronifizieren," *Der Nervenarzt* 3 (1999): 225–232.

7. Jürgen Krämer, "Presidential Address: Natural Course and Prognosis of Intervertebral Disc Disease," *Spine* 20 (1995): 635–639.

8. Richard Deyo, "Low-Back Pain," *Scientific American*, August 1998.

9. Ibid.

10. Heger, 225–232.

11. Richard Deyo and James Weinstein, "Low Back Pain," *New England Journal of Medicine* 344 (2001): 363–370.

12. Ingrid Gralow, "Psychosoziale Risikofaktoren in der Chronifizierung von Rückenschmerzen," *Schmerz* 14 (2000): 104–110.

13. Jan Hildebrandt, "Die Muskulatur als Ursache für Rückenschmerzen," *Schmerz* 17 (2003): 412–418.

14. Ibid.

15. Michael Pfingsten and Jan Hildebrandt, "Die Behandlung Chronischer Rückenschmerzen durch ein Intensives Aktivierungskonzept (GRIP)—Eine Bilanz von 10 Jahren," *Anästhesiol Intensivmed Notfallmed Schmerzther* 36 (2001): 580–589.

16. Kolata.

17. Michael Strumpf and others, "Medikamentöse Therapie bei Rückenschmerzen," *Schmerz* 15 (2001): 453–460.

18. Pfingsten and Hildebrandt, 580–589.

19. James Weinstein and others, "Surgical Versus Nonoperative Treatment for Lumbar Disk Herniation," *Journal of the American Medical Association* 296 (2006): 2441–2450.

20. Eugene Carragee, "Surgical Treatment of Lumbar Disk Disorders," *Journal of the American Medical Association* 296 (2006): 2485–2487.

21. Jeremy Fairbank and others, "Randomised Controlled Trial to Compare Surgical Stabilisation of the Lumbar Spine with an Intensive Rehabilitation Programme for Patients with Chronic Low Back Pain: The MRC Spine Stabilisation Trial," *British Medical Journal* 330 (2005): 1233–1238.

22. This was the mind-set at Klinikum Neustadt in Holstein, a huge German spine center, where many patients are treated after previous surgery.

23. Jens Ivar Brox and others, "Lumbar Instrumented Fusion Compared with Cognitive Intervention and Exercises in Patients with Chronic Back Pain After Previous Surgery for Disc Herniation," *Pain* 122 (2006): 145–155.

24. Ibid.

25. A. Mannion and others, "Comparison of Three Active Therapies for Chronic Low Back Pain: Results of a Randomized Clinical Trial with One-Year Follow-Up," *Rheumatology* 40 (2001): 772–778.

26. Ibid.

27. Ibid.

28. Kolata.

CHAPTER 9: EXERCISE AND BRAIN POWER

1. Wildor Hollmann and Heiko Strüder, "Gehirngesundheit, Leistungsfähigkeit und körperliche Aktivität," *Deutsche Zeitschrift für Sportmedizin* 9 (2003): 265–266.

2. Wildor Hollmann and others, "Körperliche Aktivität fördert Gehirngesundheit und Leistungsfähigkeit," *Nervenheilkunde* 9 (2003): 467–474.

3. Christine Graf and others, "Zusammenhänge zwischen Körperlicher Aktivität und Konzentration im Kindesalter—Eingangsergebnisse des CHILT-Projekts," *Deutsche Zeitschrift für Sportmedizin* 9 (2003): 242–246.

4. Claudia Voelker-Rehage, "Der Zusammenhang zwischen Motorischer und kognitiver Entwicklung im frühen Kindesalter—ein Teilergebnis der MODALIS-Studie," *Deutsche Zeitschrift für Sportmedizin* 10 (2005): 358–363.

5. Adele Diamond, "Close Interrelation of Motor Development and Cognitive Development and of the Cerebellum and Prefrontal Cortex," *Child Development* 71 (2000): 44–56.

6. A. Busche and others, "Lernen braucht Bewegung," *Praxis der Naturwissenschaften—Biologie in der Schule* 4.55 (2006): 40–44.

7. Diamond, 44–56

8. Ciba-Geigy fused in 1996 with Sandoz to become Novartis, the current manufacturer of Ritalin.

9. http://www.usdoj.gov/dea/concern/m.html, accessed October 18, 2008.

10. Nora D. Volkow and others, "Therapeutic Doses of Oral Methylphenidate Significantly Increase Extracellular Dopamine in the Human Brain," *The Journal of Neuroscience* 21 (2001): 1–5, reprint at: www.jneurosci.org/cgi/reprint/21/2/RC121.

11. Personal communication, March 2, 2007.

12. Diamond, 44–56.

13. Personal communication, February 19, 2007.

14. Personal communication, Christina Hahn, March 2, 2007.

CHAPTER 10: LIFTING THE SPIRIT

1. Andreas Broocks, "Körperliches Training in der Behandlung psychischer Erkrankungen," *Bundesgesundheitsbl—Gesundheitsforsch—Gesundheitsschutz* 8 (2005): 914–921.

2. Norbert-Ullrich Neumann and Karel Frasch, "Biologische Mechanismen antidepressiver Wirksamkeit von körperlicher Aktivität," *Psychoneuro* 31 (2005): 513–517.

3. Broocks, 914–921.

4. Michael Babyak and others, "Exercise Treatment for Major Depression: Maintenance of Therapeutic Benefit at 10 Months," *Psychosomatic Medicine* 62 (2000): 633–638.

5. Compare to the press release from the DukeMed news office on October 24, 1999: "Exercise May Be Just as Effective as Medication for Treating Major Depression."

6. Andrea Dunn and others, "Exercise Treatment for Depression," *American Journal of Preventive Medicine* 28 (2005): 1–8.

7. Broocks, 914–921.

8. Ibid.

9. The Latin proverb about the sound mind in a sound body (mens sana in corpore sano) is a truncated quotation that took on a life of its own. Juvenal actually said that—rather than for wealth, power, or children—men should *pray* for a sound mind in a sound body.

10. Paul A. Adlard and others, "Voluntary Exercise Decreases Amyloid Load in a Transgenic Model of Alzheimer's Disease," *The Journal of Neuroscience* 25.17 (April 27, 2005): 4217–4221.

11. Shari Roan, "To Keep the Brain Sharp, Hone the Body," *Los Angeles Times*, February 6, 2006.

12. Norbert-Ullrich Neumann and Karel Frasch: "Prävention und Therapie demenzieller Erkrankungen mittels körperlicher Akivität," *Krankenhauspsychiatrie* 17 (2006): 155–159.

13. Robert Abbott and others, "Walking and Dementia in Physically Capable Elderly Men," *Journal of the American Medical Association* 292 (2004): 1447–1453.

14. Suvi Rovio and others, "Leisure-Time Physical Activity at Midlife and the Risk of Dementia and Alzheimer's Disease," *Lancet Neurology* 4 (2005): 705–711.

15. Stanley Colcombe and others, "Aerobic Exercise Training Increases Brain Volume in Aging Humans," *Journal of Gerontology* 61A (2006): 1166–1170.

16. Ibid.

CHAPTER 11: A FOUNTAIN OF YOUTH IN THE BRAIN

1. Personal communication. Jeffrey Macklis granted me an interview on March 30, 2006, in his lab at Massachusetts General Hospital, originally reported in *Der Spiegel* magazine number 20 (2006).

2. Elkhonon Goldberg granted me an interview on March 22, 2006, in Manhattan for my reporting in *Der Spiegel* magazine number 20 (2006). His book *The Wisdom Paradox* was published in the United States and the United Kingdom.

3. Gerd Kempermann, *Adult Neurogenesis* (Oxford: Oxford University Press, 2006).

4. Ana Pereira and others, "An In Vivo Correlate of Exercise-Induced Neurogenesis in the Adult Dentate Gyrus," *Proceedings of the National Academy of Sciences of the United States of America* 104 (2007): 5638–5643.

5. Henriette van Praag, Gerd Kempermann, and Fred Gage, "Running Increases Cell Proliferation and Neurogenesis in the Adult Mouse Dentate Gyrus," *Nature Neuroscience* 2 (1999): 266–270.

6. Henriette van Praag and others, "Exercise Enhances Learning and Hippocampal Neurogenesis in Aged Mice," *The Journal of Neuroscience* 25 (2005): 8680–8685.

7. Ibid.

8. Johannes Thome and Amelia Eisch, "Neuroneogenese," *Der Nervenarzt* 76 (2005): 11–19.

9. Michael Specter, "Rethinking the Brain," *The New Yorker*, July 23, 2001.

10. Personal communication, March 2006.

11. Thome and Eisch, 11–19.

12. Jean Marx, "Preventing Alzheimer's: A Lifelong Commitment?" *Science* 309 (2005): 864–866.

13. Ibid.

14. Heather A. Lindstrom and others, "The Relationships Between Television Viewing in Midlife and the Development of Alzheimer's Disease in a Case-Control Study," *Brain and Cognition* 58 (2005): 157–165.

15. Ibid.

16. Martin Lövdén and others, "Social Participation Attenuates Decline in Perceptual Speed in Old and Very Old Age," *Psychology and Aging* 20 (2005): 423–434.

CHAPTER 12: CANCER: A GROWING CASE FOR EXERCISE

1. Anne McTiernan and others, "Effect of a 12-Month Exercise Intervention on Patterns of Cellular Proliferation in Colonic Crypts: A

Randomized Controlled Trial," *Cancer Epidemiology, Biomarkers & Prevention* 15.9 (2006): 1588–1597.

2. Petra Lahmann and others, "Physical Activity and Breast Cancer Risk: The European Prospective Investigation into Cancer and Nutrition," *Cancer Epidemiology, Biomarkers & Prevention* 10.1158/doi: 1055–9965.EPI-06–0582, published online December 19, 2006.

3. Kim Westerlind, "Physical Activity and Cancer Prevention—Mechanisms," *Medicine and Science in Sports and Exercise* 35 (2003): 1834–1840.

4. Anne McTiernan and others, "Relation of BMI and Physical Activity to Sex Hormones in Postmenopausal Women," *Obesity* 14 (2006): 1662–1677.

5. www.fhcrc.org/about/pubs/center_news/2006/oct19/art1.html.

6. These proteins are called sex hormone binding globuline (SHBG).

7. Inger Gram, Ellen Funkhouser, and Laszlo Tabar, "Moderate Physical Activity in Relation to Mammographic Patterns," *Cancer Epidemiology, Biomarkers & Prevention* 8 (1999): 117–122.

8. "Writing Group for the Women's Health Initiative Investigators: Risks and Benefits of Estrogen Plus Progestin in Healthy Postmenopausal Women," *Journal of the American Medical Association* 288 (2002): 321–333.

9. L. Hoffman-Goetz and others, "Effect of 17 Beta-Estradiol and Voluntary Exercise on Lymphocyte Apoptosis in Mice," *Physiology & Behavior* 74 (2001): 653–658.

10. Westerlind, 1834–1840.

11. Robert S. Mazzeo, "The Influence of Exercise and Aging on Immune Function," *Medicine and Science in Sports and Exercise* 26.5 (1994): 586–592.

12. Westerlind, 1834–1840.

13. Andrew G. Renehan and others, "Body-Mass Index and Incidence of Cancer: A Systematic Review and Meta-Analysis of Prospective Observational Studies," *The Lancet* 371 (2008): 569–578.

14. Zhihong Gong and others, "Obesity, Diabetes, and Risk of Prostate Cancer: Results from the Prostate Cancer Prevention Trial," *Cancer Epidemiology, Biomarkers & Prevention* 15 (2006): 1977–1983.

15. Thomas Hawighorst and Günter Emons, "Adipositas und Krebs," *Der Gynäkologe* 12 (2006): 975–980.

16: Eugenia E. Calle and others, "Overweight, Obesity, and Mortality from Cancer in a Prospectively Studied Cohort of U.S. Adults," *New England Journal of Medicine* 348 (2003): 1625–1638.

17. Kristin Campbell and Anne McTiernan, "Exercise and Biomarkers for Cancer Prevention Studies," *The Journal of Nutrition* 137 (2007): 161S–169S.

18. Hawighorst and Emons, 975–980.

19. Westerlind, 1834–1840.

20. Personal communication, Freerk Baumann, Institute for Rehabilitation at the German Sport University in Cologne, January 23, 2007.

21. Fernando Dimeo, "Welche Rolle Spielt körperliche Aktivität in der Prävention, Therapie und Rehabilitation von neoplastischen Erkrankungen?" *Deutsche Zeitschrift für Sportmedizin* 7/8 (2004): 177–182.

22. Anna Schwartz and others, "Exercise Reduces Daily Fatigue in Women with Breast Cancer Receiving Chemotherapy," *Medicine and Science in Sports and Exercise* 33.5 (2001): 718–723; see also Anna Schwartz, "Exercise and Weight Gain in Breast Cancer Patients Receiving Chemotherapy," *Cancer Practice* 8.5 (2000): 231–237.

23. Anna Schwartz: *Cancer Fitness: Exercise Programs for Patients and Survivors* (Riverside, N.J.: Simon & Schuster, 2004).

24. John Horn, "Like Lance, They Live and Ride Strong," *Los Angeles Times*, October 3, 2005.

25. Margaret McNeely and others, "Effect of Exercise on Breast Cancer Patients and Survivors: A Systematic Review and Meta-Analysis," *Canadian Medical Association Journal* 175.1 (2006): 34–41.

26. Tetsuya Ohira and others. "Effects of Weight Training on Quality of Life in Recent Breast Cancer Survivors. The Weight Training for Breast Cancer Survivors (WTBS) Study," *Cancer* 106 (2006): 2076–2083.

27. Press release of the University of Texas M. D. Anderson Cancer Center in Houston, July 17, 2006.

28. Freeke Baumann and others, "Auswirkungen von Bewegungs-therapien bei und nach Knochenmark-/Stammzelltransplantation," *Deutsche Zeitschrift für Onkologie* 37.4 (2005): 152–158.

29. Jeffrey Meyerhardt and others, "Impact of Physical Activity on Cancer Recurrence and Survival in Patients with Stage III Colon Cancer: Findings from CALGB 89803," *Journal of Clinical Oncology* 24.22 (2006): 3535–3541.

30. Jeffrey Meyerhardt and others, "Physical Activity and Survival After Colorectal Cancer Diagnosis," *Journal of Clinical Oncology* 24 (2006): 3527–3534.

31. Michelle Holmes and others, "Physical Activity and Survival after Breast Cancer Diagnosis," *Journal of the American Medical Association* 293.20 (2005): 2479–2486.

32. www.cancer.gov/newscenter/pressreleases/herceptinCombination 2005.

33. Wendy Demark-Wahnefried, "Cancer Survival: Time to Get Moving? Data Accumulate Suggesting a Link Between Physical Activity and Cancer Survival," *Journal of Clinical Oncology* 24.22 (2006): 3517–3518.

CHAPTER 13: LONGEVITY, POTENCY, AND RESILIENCE

1. http://en.wikipedia.org/wiki/Life_expectancy.

2. 78.14 years in 2008 (estimated according to https://www.cia.gov/library/publications/the-world-factbook/index.html.

3. Steven Rosenberg, "Oh, the Things You Will See if You Live to Be 110," *The Boston Globe*, February 16, 2006.

4. Jeremiah Barondess, "On the Preservation of Health," *Journal of the American Medical Association* 294 (2005): 3024–3026.

5. If humans are born to run, one might wonder why some runners have problems with their knees. Daniel Lieberman of Harvard University says that our forebears never ran on a hard surface such as concrete or asphalt. Furthermore, today's runner wears shoes that actually weakens the muscles and joints, thus making them prone for wear and tear. Finally, our forebears were not obese. Dennis Bramble and Daniel

Lieberman, "Endurance Running and the Evolution of Homo," *Nature* 432 (2004): 345–352.

6. *The Boston Globe*, March 23, 2007.

7. Urho M. Kujala and others, "Relationship of Leisure-Time Physical Activity and Mortality," *Journal of the American Medical Association* 279 (1998): 440–444; reprint at http://jama.ama-assn.org/cgi/reprint/279/6/440.pdf.

8. The genetic component for cardiovascular diseases is estimated to be 30 percent; Herbert Löllgen and Deborah Löllgen, "Körperliche Aktivität und Primärprävention," *Deutsche Medizinische Wochenschrift* 129 (2004): 1055–1056; reprint at www.thieme-connect.com/ejournals/pdf/dmw/doi/10.1055/s-2004–824858.pdf.

9. John Hoberman and Charles Yesalis, "The History of Synthetic Testosterone," *Scientific American*, February 1995.

10. K. Sreekumaran Nair and others, "DHEA in Elderly Women and DHEA or Testosterone in Elderly Men," *New England Journal of Medicine* 355 (2006): 1647–1659.

11. Henry Feldman and others, "Age Trends in the Level of Serum Testosterone and Other Hormones in Middle-Aged Men: Longitudinal Results from the Massachusetts Male Aging Study," *The Journal of Clinical Endocrinology and Metabolism* 87 (2002): 589–598.

12. Thomas Travison and others, "The Relative Contributions of Aging, Health, and Lifestyle Factors to Serum Testosterone Decline in Men," *The Journal of Clinical Endocrinology and Metabolism* 92 (2007): 549–555.

13. Michael Rauchenwald, "Körperliche Fitness beim alternden Mann," *Blickpunkt Der Mann* 1 (2003): 20–23.

14. Carol Derby and others, "Modifiable Risk Factors and Erectile Dysfunction: Can Lifestyle Changes Modify Risk?" *Urology* 56 (2000): 302–306.

15. Ibid.

16. Katherine Esposito and others, "Effect of Lifestyle Changes on Erectile Dysfunction in Obese Men," *Journal of the American Medical Association* 291 (2004): 2978–2984.

17. Suresh Rattan, "Anti-Ageing Strategies: Prevention or Therapy?" *Embo Reports* 6 (2005): 25–28.

18. *Wall Street Journal* (European edition), June 24, 2006.

19. Rod Dishman and others, "Neurobiology of Exercise," *Obesity* 14 (2006): 345–356.

20. Agathocles Tsatsoulis and Stelios Fountoulakis, "The Protective Role of Exercise on Stress System Dysregulation and Comorbidities," *Annals of the New York Academy of Sciences* 1083 (2006): 196–213.

21. Jessica Chubak and others, "Moderate-Intensity Exercise Reduces the Incidence of Colds Among Postmenopausal Women," *The American Journal of Medicine* 119 (2006): 937–942.

22. Eliza F. Chakravarty and others, "Reduced Disability and Mortality Among Aging Runners," *Archives of Internal Medicine* 168.15 (2008): 1638–1646.

23. News release from Stanford University, August 20, 2008.

CHAPTER 14: PANACEA FOR EVERY DAY

1. David Bassett and others, "Physical Activity in an Old Order Amish Community," *Medicine and Science in Sports and Exercise* 36 (2004): 79–85.

2. Aloys Berg and others, "Gewichtskontrolle ist nicht nur FdH," *MMW—Fortschritte der Medizin* 27–28 (2004): 636/27–30/639.

3. Maria Fiatarone Singh, "Essay: Fit for Life—A Geriatrician's Perspective on Aging Well," *The Lancet* 366, suppl. 1 (2005): S51.

4. In yet another study Becca Levy has shown that older people who have negative stereotypes about the elderly have a greater chance of hearing decline. Levy and others, "Hearing Decline Predicted by Elders' Stereotypes," *The Journals of Gerontology, Series B, Psychological Sciences and Social Sciences* 61 (2006): 82–87; see also Gina Kolata, "Old but not Frail: A Matter of Heart and Head," *New York Times*, October 5, 2006.

5. Rainer Hambrecht and others, "Percutaneous Coronary Angioplasty Compared with Exercise Training in Patients with Stable Coro-

nary Artery Disease: A Randomized Trial," *Circulation* 109 (2004): 1371–1378.

6. There are signs suggesting the meteoric rise of angioplasty during the past three decades has ended. Interestingly, this is not because doctors started to appreciate the therapeutic value of exercise. Rather, three recent studies published in the past two years indicate that using the procedure to open blocked arteries to treat chest pain, or angina, may be riskier and no more beneficial than medication. See Steve Sternberg, "Angioplasty's Golden Era May be Fading," *USA Today*, March 26, 2008.

7. Charles Mann, "Provocative Study Says Obesity May Reduce U.S. Life Expectancy," *Science*, March 18, 2005: 1716.

8. Singh, S51.

9. News release of the Fred Hutchinson Cancer Research Center, August 4, 2008; www.fhcrc.org/about/ne/news/2008/08/04/YMCA_exercise.html.

10. www.exerciseismedicine.org, accessed October 18, 2008.

11. www.exerciseismedicine.org/media.htm, accessed October 18, 2008.

12. www.mentalhealth.org.uk/media/news-releases/news-releases-2008/8-february-2008/, accessed October 18, 2008.

13. Ralf Sygusch and others, "Gesundheitssport—Effekte und deren Nachhaltigkeit bei unterschiedlichem Energieverbrauch," *Deutsche Zeitschrift für Sportmedizin* 9 (2005): 318–326.

14. The American College of Sports Medicine (ACSM) and the American Heart Association (AHA) have jointly published physical activity guidelines. For adults over age 65 (or adults 50–64 with chronic conditions, such as arthritis), the basic recommendations are: do moderately intense aerobic exercise 30 minutes a day, five days a week; or do vigorously intense aerobic exercise 20 minutes a day, three days a week, and do 8 to 10 strength-training exercises, 10–15 repetitions of each exercise, twice to three times per week. The complete recommendations are at www.acsm.org.

15. Xuemei Sui and others, "Cardiorespiratory Fitness and Adiposity as Mortality Predictors in Older Adults," *Journal of the American Medical Association* 298 (2008): 2507–2516.

16. R. S. Pfaffenbarger and others, "Physical Activity and Physical Fitness as Determinants of Health and Longevity," in *Exercise, Fitness and Health A Consensus of Current Knowledge*, ed. C. Bouchard, R. J. Shephard, and T. Stephens (Champaign, IL: Human Kinetics, 1990), 33–48.

17. Christian Roberts and James Barnard, "Effects of Exercise and Diet on Chronic disease," *Journal of Applied Physiology* 98 (2005): 3–30.

18. *Der Spiegel* number 51 (2000).

19. www.who.int/dietphysicalactivity/publications/facts/pa/en/, accessed March 19, 2007.

20. Rainer Hambrecht and Stephan Gielen, "Essay: Hunter-Gatherer to Sedentary Lifestyle," *The Lancet* 366 (2005): S60-S61.

GUIDELINES ON THE WEB

The American College of Sports Medicine and the American Heart Association have jointly published physical activity guidelines:
www.acsm.org/AM/Template.cfm?Section=Home_Page&
TEMPLATE=/CM/HTMLDisplay.cfm&CONTENTID=7764.

The National Institute on Aging (part of the U.S. Government's National Institutes of Health) has created a comprehensive exercise program expressly with seniors in mind:
www.nia.nih.gov/HealthInformation/Publications/Exercise
Guide/.

The Surgeon General's report on physical activity and health:
www.cdc.gov/nccdphp/sgr/sgr.htm.

ACKNOWLEDGMENTS

I wish to thank Peter Dizikes, Barbara Perlmutter, and Kerstin Schuster for their help and support with this U.S. version of the book. I am particularly indebted to my editor, Merloyd Lawrence, for her suggestions and editing. I am fortunate to have met researchers and physicians who willingly shared their expertise with me: Aloys Berg, Fred Gage, Elkhonon Goldberg, Martin Halle, Christina Hahn, Rainer Hambrecht, Gertrude Huntington, Melinda Irwin, Carolyn Kaelin, Gerd Kempermann, Ulman Lindenberger, Herbert Löllgen, Jeffrey Macklis, Wilhelm Niebling, Fernando Nottebohm, Henriette van Praag, Hans-Georg Predel, Irwin Rosenberg, Robert Sallis, Eckard Schönau, Thorsten Schulz, Anna Schwartz, Heiko Strüder, Gertraud Teuchert-Noodt, Claudia Voelcker-Rehage, R. Sanders Williams, Andrea Zegelin, and Marc Ziegler.

My friend Jobst-Ulrich Brand, a journalist based in Munich, read the first version of the manuscript and provided me with valuable comments. Matthias Landwehr, my agent in Berlin, and Peter Sillem, my editor at S. Fischer in Frankfurt, encouraged me to go for this project. I am indebted to my colleagues at *Der Spiegel* magazine; Stefan Aust, Johann Grolle, and Olaf Stampf supported this project.

Most important, I wish to thank my wife and our children. They have guided me through this exciting endeavor.

INDEX

ABOUT THE AUTHOR

Jörg Blech, a native of Cologne, Germany, received his diploma in molecular biology from the University of Cologne in 1993. After studies in the Department of Chemistry and Biochemistry at the University of Sussex, England, he trained in journalism and was awarded internships in Paris, Washington DC, and Bangkok. He was science reporter for *Stern* magazine, the weekly newspaper *Die Zeit,* and since 1999 has been a staff writer at Europe's largest weekly news magazine, *Der Spiegel.* In 2005 he established the Boston bureau of *Der Spiegel* and was appointed science correspondent. His five best-selling books for a general audience have been excerpted in *Der Spiegel, Facts* magazine (Switzerland*), Profil* magazine (Austria), *El Pais* daily (Spain), *New Scientist,* and *The Guardian.* His book *Inventing Disease and Pushing Pills* has been published in a dozen languages. Jörg Blech lives with his wife and their three children in Arlington, Massachusetts.